CHRONIC RENAL FAILURE

Other titles in the *New Clinical Applications* Series:

Dermatology (Series Editor Dr J. L. Verbov)
Dermatological Surgery
Superficial Fungal Infections
Talking Points in Dermatology – I
Treatment in Dermatology
Current Concepts in Contact Dermatitis
Talking Points in Dermatology – II

Cardiology (Series Editor Dr D. Longmore)
Cardiology Screening

Rheumatology (Series Editors Dr J. J. Calabro and Dr W. Carson Dick)
Ankylosing Spondylitis
Infections and Arthritis

Nephrology (Series Editor Dr G. R. D. Catto)
Continuous Ambulatory Peritoneal Dialysis
Management of Renal Hypertension
Chronic Renal Failure
Calculus Disease
Pregnancy and Renal Disorders
Multisystem Diseases
Glomerulonephritis I
Glomerulonephritis II

NEW CLINICAL APPLICATIONS NEPHROLOGY

CHRONIC RENAL FAILURE

Editor

G. R. D. CATTO
MD, FRCP, FRCP(G)

Reader in Medicine
University of Aberdeen
UK

KLUWER ACADEMIC PUBLISHERS
DORDRECHT / BOSTON / LONDON

Distributors

for the United States and Canada: Kluwer Academic Publishers, PO Box 358, Accord Station, Hingham, MA 02018-0358, USA
for all other countries: Kluwer Academic Publishers Group, Distribution Center, PO Box 322, 3300 AH Dordrecht, The Netherlands

British Library Cataloguing in Publication Data

Chronic renal failure.
1. Man. Kidneys. Chronic renal failure
I. Catto, Graeme R. D. (Graeme Robertson Dawson), *1945–* II. Series
616.6′14

Library of Congress Cataloging-in-Publication Data

Chronic renal failure.
(New clinical applications. Nephrology)
Includes bibliographies and index.
1. Chronic renal failure. I. Catto, Graeme R. D.
II. Series. [DNLM: 1. Kidney Failure, Chronic.
WJ 342 C5572]
RC918.R4C614 1988 616.6′14 88–9277

ISBN-13: 978-94-010-7679-1 e-ISBN-13: 978-94-009-2613-4
DOI: 10.1007/978-94-009-2613-4

Published in the United Kingdom by Kluwer Academic Publishers, PO Box 55, Lancaster, UK.

Kluwer Academic Publishers BV incorporates the publishing programmes of D. Reidel, Martinus Nijhoff, Dr W. Junk and MTP Press.

CONTENTS

LIST OF AUTHORS

G. A. Coles
KRUF Institute of Renal Disease
University of Wales College of Medicine
Cardiff Royal Infirmary
Newport Road, Cardiff CF2 1SZ
UK

A. J. Felsenfeld
Nephrology Section
University of Oklahoma Health Sciences Center and VAMC
Oklahoma City, Oklahoma 73104
USA

F. Llach
Nephrology Section
University of Oklahoma Health Sciences Center and VAMC
Oklahoma City, Oklahoma 73104
USA

N. Muirhead
Department of Nephrology/Medicine
University of Western Ontario
London, Ontario N6A 5A5
Canada

A. V. Murphy
Renal Unit
Royal Hospital for Sick Children
Yorkhill
Glasgow G3 8SJ
UK

SERIES EDITOR'S FOREWORD

For the last two decades, the topic of chronic renal failure has been dominated by discussions on dialysis and transplantation. As facilities for treating patients with end-stage renal failure have become more readily available, at least in Europe and North America, attention has once again been drawn to conservative measures which may improve both the overall prognosis and the quality of life of patients with renal impairment. Although severe renal failure may be progressive and many patients will ultimately require some form of renal replacement therapy, it is now widely appreciated that distressing symptoms can often be ameliorated by judicious medical treatment. Children as well as, and perhaps to a greater extent than, adults may benefit from such therapy.

This volume examines relevant trends in the conservative management of both adults and children with chronic renal failure. Each chapter has been written by recognized experts and provides information of clinical relevance for the average clinician. As the overall prognosis for patients with end-stage renal failure improves it is clear the management of patients with relatively stable chronic renal failure is an important topic not only for nephrologists but for all practising clinicians.

G. R. D. Catto

ABOUT THE EDITOR

Dr Graeme R. D. Catto is Reader in Medicine at the University of Aberdeen and Honorary Consultant Physician/Nephrologist to the Grampian Health Board. His current interest in transplant immunology was stimulated as a Harkness Fellow at Harvard Medical School and the Peter Bent Brigham Hospital, Boston, USA. He is a member of many medical societies including the Association of Physicians of Great Britain and Ireland, the Renal Association and the Transplantation Society. He has published widely on transplant and reproductive immunology, calcium metabolism and general nephrology.

1

NUTRITIONAL MANAGEMENT OF CHRONIC RENAL FAILURE

G. A. COLES

INTRODUCTION

Nutrition plays a key role in chronic renal failure. In advanced uraemia the symptoms of anorexia, nausea and vomiting inevitably mean that the intake of nutrients is suboptimal. An additional cause of reduced food consumption is the widespread use of low protein diets for symptomatic treatment of this condition. It is therefore not surprising that numerous studies have shown that varying degrees of malnutrition are common in patients with chronic renal failure. It is perhaps more disturbing to discover that patients treated by long-term dialysis also have evidence of undernutrition[1,2].

The range of abnormalities described includes disturbances of body composition, low serum protein levels, altered amino acid metabolism, depletion of vitamins and metals and reduction of body fat and muscle mass. Thus it is likely that part of the uraemic syndrome may well be due to malnutrition. It is clearly desirable that patients be maintained in as optimal a nutritional state as possible. This aim has become even more important with the recent suggestion that a low nitrogen intake may slow the progression of chronic renal failure and should be used in individuals who are still asymptomatic.

This chapter reviews the evidence for protein-calorie depletion in chronic uraemia and considers ways of assessing nutritional status. The nutritional requirements at different stages of the illness are discussed and the possible influence of diet on progression of human renal failure is reviewed. Finally, methods for assessing dietary compliance are detailed.

NUTRITIONAL PROBLEMS IN CHRONIC RENAL FAILURE

Body composition

Several studies using mainly isotope dilution techniques have shown that a significant proportion of patients with chronic renal failure have abnormalities of body composition[3,4]. These changes are commonest in subjects with advanced disease who have not received dialysis.

Body weight is often reduced below expected values for height due to losses of body fat (as assessed by skinfold thickness) and fat-free solids. Lean body mass forms an increased proportion of body weight. Total body water is relatively increased mainly due to excess extracellular fluid. Intracellular fluid is reduced in relation to expected or standard weight, though occasional individuals may have an increased intracellular volume as well as extracellular expansion. Exchangeable sodium is often greater than normal but total body potassium tends to be reduced. These changes are interpreted as meaning there is loss of body fat and also cellular tissue in many patients with chronic renal failure, with an expansion of extracellular fluid.

Following the start of long-term haemodialysis, body weight tends to fall due to a loss of water, mostly from the extracellular compartment, even in patients without overt oedema. Body fat increases and some patients may gain fat-free solids. Despite these changes a proportion of patients continue to have an excess extracellular fluid and a reduced intracellular space. Following intercurrent illness the abnormalities found in untreated advanced uraemia rapidly recur.

During continuous ambulatory peritoneal dialysis (CAPD) body fat increases and some patients have a rise in lean body mass. A major component of the lean body mass is muscle. Muscle mass can be assessed from arm muscle circumference and several surveys have shown that a proportion of patients with chronic renal failure have abnormally low values for this measurement. This finding has been noted in subjects receiving haemodialysis, CAPD or just conservative treatment.

Similar changes in body composition have been well documented in subjects suffering from simple malnutrition. Although there are abnormalities of sodium and water handling by the kidney in renal failure and intermittent excess of intake during dialysis treatment, it seems likely that many of these changes are caused by protein-calorie deficiency, due to either an inadequate diet or failure of intake by the patient.

Figure 1.1 shows the typical body composition changes of a patient with advanced renal failure as compared to a normal subject.

Proteins and amino acids

Reduced serum proteins, particularly albumin and transferrin, are a common finding in uraemia[5]. Non-dialysed chronic renal failure patients as a group have statistically lower values for these two proteins compared to healthy individuals and a considerable number have

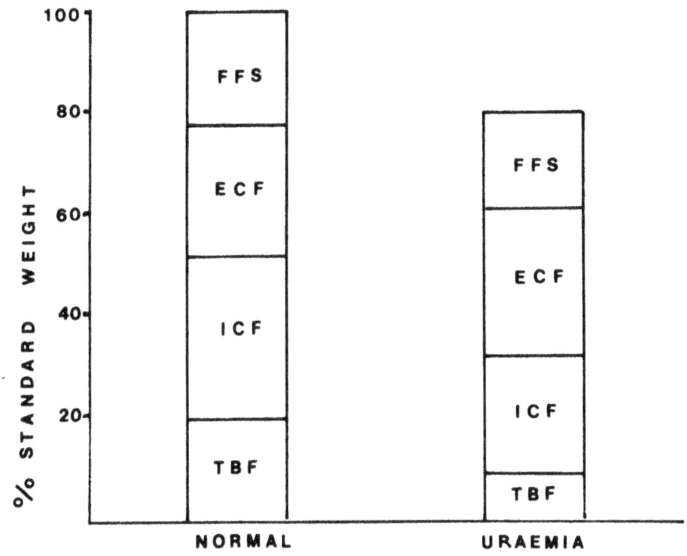

FIGURE 1.1 Comparison of body composition in a normal subject to that of a patient with chronic uraemia. ECF = extracellular fluid; ICF = intracellular fluid; FFS = fat-free solids; TBF = total body fat. Total body water (TBW) = ECF + ICF. Lean body mass = TBW + FFS

subnormal levels. Following the start of haemodialysis, serum albumin tends to return to within the normal range[6]. During CAPD treatment, however, many patients have somewhat reduced values.

The reduction in serum proteins is in part due to external losses. Some patients, despite advanced renal failure, may continue to pass nephrotic range amounts of protein in the urine, i.e. 5 g or more per 24 hours. During haemodialysis approximately 5–8 g of free amino acids and 3–4 g of bound amino acids are removed during a 4-hour treatment. CAPD is associated with losses of approximately 8 g of protein per 24 hours as well as 2 g of amino acids. However, during peritonitis the amount of protein lost in the dialysate rapidly increases and is reflected in a considerable fall in serum albumin levels. A similar drop may occur in haemodialysis patients who suffer an intercurrent illness.

Albumin metabolism has been investigated in stable non-dialysed uraemic individuals[6]. They have a reduced total albumin mass particularly due to a reduction in the extravascular pool. Albumin synthesis and catabolism are often reduced. Identical abnormalities are found in subjects with protein-calorie malnutrition and thus these findings confirm that protein depletion is common in individuals with chronic renal failure. Whether this depletion is solely due to a reduced protein intake is still not entirely clear. Patients on haemodialysis tend to have normal catabolic rates[7]. During intercurrent illness catabolism may increase considerably but falls to normal when the patient recovers. Subjects undergoing CAPD may have a normal total albumin mass. Catabolism appears to be reduced but synthesis is increased correlating with the amount lost in the dialysate[8].

Muscle

Muscle forms the body's largest store of protein. As already noted patients may have a reduced muscle mass as assessed by anthropometry and a low total body potassium. One study has suggested that CAPD patients have a reduced total body nitrogen probably reflecting some loss of muscle protein. However, due to methodological problems there are no reliable measurements of muscle protein synthesis and degradation in subjects with chronic renal failure. Examination of muscle biopsies from such individuals has shown a reduced content of non-collagenous protein and RNA in relation to DNA, suggesting that intracellular protein stores and the capacity for protein synthesis were reduced[9].

In chronic uraemic rats myofibrillar degradation is increased even when the animals are fed. On fasting the uraemic animals have a lower muscle protein synthesis and higher degradation than controls of the same weight[10]. This abnormal response to stress appears to be related to reduced energy stores. In patients this reduction may be reflected in the low body fat.

Amino acids

Patients with chronic renal failure have an abnormal pattern of amino acids in their sera[11]. The essential amino acids, threonine, valine, leucine, lysine, histidine and tyrosine, are reduced together with the non-essential serine. Methionine and phenylalanine tend to be raised as are the non-essential amino acids, aspartic acid, glutamic acid, citrulline, ornithine and arginine.

Intracellular levels of amino acids as judged by muscle biopsy analysis are also abnormal in uraemia, but the pattern is different from plasma. There is a low concentration of valine, threonine, lysine and histidine, but normal values for leucine and isoleucine. Protein synthesis depends on having the essential amino acids in the correct proportions inside the cell. Since in renal failure some of these are reduced, their availability will limit the capacity for protein formation. The surplus remaining amino acids may well be catabolized for energy adding to the nitrogen load.

Some of these amino acid abnormalities are nutritional in origin since the majority return to normal in the intracellular compartment when patients are well fed and treated by haemodialysis. Similarly, the taking of specially formulated amino acid preparations can correct some of the findings. However, high levels of phenylalanine, citrulline, ornithine and arginine tend to persist, suggesting that they are caused by the uraemic process itself.

Carbohydrate

Carbohydrate intolerance is a well-recognized abnormality in chronic uraemia[12]. Fasting blood glucose levels are normal or slightly increased and fasting insulin concentrations are normal or raised. However, there is an impaired response to a glucose load. The main reason for this finding is tissue insensitivity, particularly muscle, to insulin. The exact nature of this resistance is uncertain. Insulin appears to bind normally to monocytes from uraemic subjects so the problem may be due to a post-binding intracellular defect. Raised circulating levels of glucagon and growth hormone may also contribute to the abnormal glucose metabolism.

On its own the carbohydrate intolerance is of little clinical importance but it may have other consequences. There could be increased glycosylation of structural proteins. Haemoglobin A_1 levels are raised in uraemia. However, recent work has shown that this is due to increased carbamylation due to high levels of blood urea. Specific glycosylated haemoglobin is not raised in chronic renal failure except in diabetics. The insulin resistance might also contribute to hypertriglyceridaemia. Insulin is an important regulator of lipoprotein lipase which controls the removal of triglycerides from the circulation. It is unclear whether uraemic insulin antagonism affects the activity of this enzyme.

Neither dialysis nor a low-protein diet corrects the carbohydrate intolerance. Thus the abnormality is probably directly related to the uraemic state and not the patient's nutrition.

CAPD treatment leads to the absorption of dextrose in considerable quantities contributing to hyperinsulinaemia. During peritonitis this absorption is often enhanced and leads to loss of ultrafiltration since the osmotic gradient is rapidly abolished[13]. Occasional patients develop frank diabetes mellitus probably because the absorbed dextrose is too great for the endogenous insulin.

Lipids

Most uraemic patients have a normal total cholesterol concentration but a significant proportion varying from a third to a half have raised fasting triglycerides. Study of the lipoprotein classes reveals that there is an increase in very low density lipoprotein (VLDL) and sometimes low density lipoprotein (LDL), together with a decrease in high density lipoprotein (HDL)[12]. Most reports indicate that impaired catabolism rather than increased production is responsible for the raised triglyceride levels[14]. Post-heparin lipolytic activity in the plasma and hepatic lipoprotein lipase are both reduced. More recently, adipose tissue lipoprotein lipase has also been found to be reduced and fails to increase after a meal in patients with hypertriglyceridaemia.

Individuals treated by haemodialysis have a similar range of abnormalities. Patients receiving CAPD may be exposed to large quantities of dextrose and tend to have rising triglycerides, VLDL and total cholesterol, whereas HDL and LDL remain constant[15]. Those subjects who avoid using the more hypertonic bags are less likely to develop hyperlipidaemia.

Other factors which may contribute to the observed lipid changes include a possible deficiency of carnitine[16]. This compound is concerned in the intracellular transport of fatty acids to the oxidative site in the mitochondria. During dialysis treatment plasma levels of carnitine fall. However, there is still controversy as to the contribution that any deficiency may make to the changes in plasma lipids seen in chronic renal failure[17].

Though it is likely that the uraemic process plays a part in producing the altered lipids, nutrition also seems to be a factor since decreasing the calories derived from carbohydrates and increasing the polyunsaturated to saturated fatty acid ratio to 1:1 has been reported to result in a lowering of the triglycerides to normal[18,19]. It is noteworthy that exercise training is also recorded as producing the same effect.

The abnormalities described in chronic renal failure are associated with an increased risk of atherosclerosis in non-uraemic individuals. Whether correcting these changes in patients with chronic uraemia reduces the chances of vascular disease is still uncertain.

Vitamins and metals

There is a tendency for patients with chronic renal failure to develop deficiencies of water-soluble vitamins[20]. This is particularly likely to occur in those individuals on a very restricted intake, either prescribed by the clinician or due to the symptoms of uraemia itself. There may also be losses of water-soluble vitamins during a dialysis treatment. Patients who are on a low potassium but normal protein diet may well have a low vitamin C intake due to a reduced allowance of fruit and vegetables in the menu and the need to double boil potatoes. However, there is still controversy as to whether any such deficiencies are clinically significant. There is some biochemical evidence suggesting that low vitamin B_6 (pyridoxine) levels limit the activity of erythrocyte glutamic pyruvic transaminase in uraemia[21]. Patients have been described as having reduced plasma and leukocyte ascorbic acid levels. Though there has been one report of mild clinical scurvy, this has not been noted by most clinicians. Occasional patients appear to become folate depleted but the majority do not develop this problem.

Recent work suggests that many subjects receiving haemodialysis maintain their plasma vitamin levels without any need for supplements[22]. A few individuals tend to have low values for pyridoxine, folate, thiamine and niacin. Vitamin B_{12}, though water soluble, is not easily lost by dialysis, probably because it binds to protein. Thus B_{12} deficiency is not a problem for uraemic patients.

The fat-soluble vitamins do not appear to be deficient in chronic renal failure with the exception of vitamin D whose renal metabolism is considerably reduced. Vitamin A levels are raised as is the concentration of retinol-binding protein. There also appears to be an increased content of vitamin A in the liver. Vitamin E levels have been reported to be reduced, normal or even raised in uraemic patients but the clinical significance of any abnormalities remains uncertain. No alteration of vitamin K metabolism has been reported in chronic renal failure.

A low protein intake will usually involve a reduction in the consumption of various metals, in particular calcium, iron and zinc. This is especially likely to occur if protein ingestion falls below $0.5 g\,kg^{-1}\,day^{-1}$. Maintaining an adequate calcium intake is important in the prevention and management of renal osteodystrophy.

Patients receiving haemodialysis frequently develop iron deficiency because of the inevitable blood losses involved in this treatment. Inadequate iron consumption can also produce the same clinical effect. Iron absorption appears to be normal in uraemia.

Total body zinc is apparently increased in chronic renal failure but plasma and muscle concentrations are reduced implying that a redistribution of this metal has occurred[23]. Despite this rise in whole body levels there still appears to be a relative deficiency of zinc in some tissues, since supplementing the diet has been reported to improve taste and appetite and thus nutrition in general. Initially, it was claimed that zinc improved uraemic impotence but this has not been confirmed.

Total body rubidium is considerably reduced in chronic renal failure, more so than potassium. The clinical significance is still uncertain.

Consequences of uraemic malnutrition

For thousands of years it has been recognized that severe or extreme malnutrition is associated with serious morbidity and death, often due to infection. However, only a small minority of chronic renal failure patients are seen with gross emaciation. The question arises as to whether the lesser degrees of malnutrition, commonly found in uraemic individuals, are of any serious clinical significance. Some of the clinical and laboratory features of uraemia are similar to those produced by protein-calorie deficiency. It has therefore been difficult to determine what abnormalities are directly due to the uraemic state, with its retention of metabolites and abnormal metabolism, or due to associated malnutrition. For instance, there is depressed cell-mediated immunity in both conditions but it is still not clear whether the improvement seen with dialysis treatment represents correction of the uraemic state with possible removal of potential inhibitors, a better nutritional state or a combination of both.

It has been well established that hospitalized patients in general, who have significant degrees of malnutrition, have a worse prognosis and are more likely to suffer infection than normal individuals[24]. Although there are few studies comparing nutrition and outcome in uraemic subjects, it has been reported that both haemodialysis[25] and

CAPD patients[26] who have a low serum albumin have a higher incidence of infection.

There is evidence that patients who are serially followed by a renal unit and started on dialysis when they become symptomatic have a significantly better prognosis than those subjects who are referred late and require to start replacement therapy almost immediately. It is likely that part of the difference is due to a worse nutritional state in the late referral group, though no firm data are available to confirm or refute this suggestion.

Haemodialysis subjects with a relatively low body mass index, the relation of weight to the square of height, appear to have a higher mortality than other patients[27]. Furthermore, individuals having malnutrition as judged by reduced relative body weight, anthropometric measurements or serum albumin appeared to have a higher mortality than those judged as normal when followed up on haemodialysis for more than 3 years[28]. In this author's own experience patients starting haemodialysis with a weight less than 75% of standard weight had a significantly greater mortality during the first 6 months of treatment than those whose weight was higher. It is of interest that in all these studies cardiovascular disease has been the commonest cause of death rather than infection. The nature of the relationship, if any, between uraemic malnutrition and cardiovascular disease is uncertain.

Recently, it has been found that chronic renal failure patients who are well nourished have normal muscle function compared to controls. Uraemic subjects with objective evidence of malnutrition had significantly worse function than either of the other groups[29]. Thus nutrition rather than uraemia *per se* appears to influence muscle performance in this clinical situation. Lymphocyte function correlates with nutritional status in patients having haemodialysis. Clearly, in those small numbers of uraemic patients who develop a megaloblastic anaemia from folic acid depletion, there is a direct link between nutrition and the clinical picture.

Although many patients have only a relatively mild degree of protein-calorie deficiency, this state may rapidly worsen if there is any intercurrent illness. Chronic uraemic individuals rapidly become anorexic when ill so that nutritional intake becomes inadequate. In certain conditions, e.g. peritonitis or other sepsis, there may be direct depletion of protein. In these situations unless prompt treatment is instituted the degree of malnutrition will rapidly become serious.

In conclusion, when considering the consequences of malnutrition in chronic renal failure, the evidence that is available together with the information obtained from non-uraemic individuals strongly suggests that neglecting the nutritional status of uraemic patients may predispose to increased morbidity and mortality.

ASSESSMENT OF NUTRITION

Since the nutritional status of patients with chronic renal failure is of clinical significance, it is important to assess the degree of any protein-calorie depletion. Numerous techniques have been used but many are not suitable for routine purposes. Body composition measurements require the use of isotope dilution techniques or, in the case of total body potassium, a whole body counter. Total body nitrogen can be quantified but only by the complex technique of neutron activation analysis. In non-renal patients urinary creatinine excretion correlates well with muscle mass. Unfortunately, in chronic renal failure an increasing proportion of the endogenous creatinine disappears from the plasma by one or more non-renal routes and thus urinary measurement underestimates true creatinine production. Muscle biopsy analysis correlates well with whole body changes but is too invasive for routine usage. Measurements of albumin turnover are similarly not suitable for widespread application. There are, however, a few standard techniques which can be easily applied to any patient[1,30–32].

Weight

Changes in body weight provide the simplest method of assessing nutrition. Comparison is made to values in published tables for the same height and sex, sometimes called the standard weight. Patients, who when first seen are more than 10% below their standard weight, are at risk of having malnutrition. Clearly, a falling weight means the nutritional status is deteriorating, but a steady or even normal value does not exclude serious deficiency.

As already noted, patients starting on dialysis may not have obvious oedema but their degree of overhydration becomes apparent as they lose fluid during each dialysis session. It follows that fluid retention may well mask a decline in dry body weight. It is therefore essential to determine a patient's true dry weight, particularly after starting dialysis as one means of assessing the degree of any malnutrition. Dry weight in this clinical context is defined as the minimum value obtained in the absence of hypotension.

Serum proteins

A number of serum proteins have been used in the assessment of patients' nutrition. In particular the concentration of albumin has been extensively investigated as an aid to the diagnosis of malnutrition. Subnormal levels correlate with increased morbidity and mortality in all types of patient including those with renal failure. Unfortunately, a normal value does not exclude nutritional depletion. If undernutrition does not occur rapidly there is first a reduction in extravascular albumin mass before the intravascular mass starts to fall. Studies on patients with chronic renal failure show that a reduced extravascular albumin mass with a normal serum concentration occurs quite frequently. Furthermore, serum albumin can also be maintained when muscle mass, as assessed by anthropometry, is declining. Thus a reduced concentration is a relatively late indication of malnutrition.

Transferrin has been suggested as being more suitable as a marker of protein-calorie depletion. Patients with chronic uraemia are reported to have statistically lower serum concentrations than normal controls, but many individuals have levels within the normal range. Again serum transferrin can be steady in the face of decreasing muscle mass.

Pre-albumin and retinol binding protein have much shorter half-lives than either albumin or transferrin and thus their concentrations should reflect recent nutritional changes much better. This seems to be true in non-renal subjects but unfortunately the levels of both proteins are raised in uraemia, invalidating their usage as markers of protein depletion.

Anthropometry

Anthropometry means direct measurement of part of the human body. In the context of nutrition two parameters are in widespread use – namely skinfold thickness as an assessment of body fat and muscle circumference representing the body's protein stores.

Body fat provides the reserve pool of energy during starvation. Subcutaneous fat forms a large proportion (approximately 50%) of the adipose tissue and thus changes in the amount of subcutaneous fat reflect whole body variations. When a skinfold is produced by gentle pinching most of its thickness is due to the subdermal adipose tissue. Various sites have been suggested for measuring skinfold thickness and there are formulae in existence for calculating body fat in kilograms from the observed values. In routine clinical practice this is not necessary. For ease and simplicity a single site, the triceps skinfold, is usually chosen. It is important to use a calliper which provides a constant pressure on the skin irrespective of the gap between the jaws. Usually the non-dominant or, on haemodialysis subjects, the non-fistula arm is chosen. The method is subject to error but if measurements are taken in triplicate by the same observer at the same point, it becomes reproducible. Tables have been published of normal values but the technique is of most value for following serial changes in an individual.

Mid-arm muscle circumference (MAMC) is derived from mid-arm circumference (MAC) measured with a tape measure and the triceps skinfold thickness (TSF) at the same point on the arm, using the formula

$$\text{MAMC} = \text{MAC} - (\pi \times \text{TSF})$$

The area enclosed in the MAMC consists mostly of muscle and bone. Bone area is assumed to be relatively constant in adults and thus changes in MAMC represent alteration in muscle mass, i.e. a large proportion of the body's protein stores. Once again, serial measurements on an individual are of more value than a single assessment except when there is severe malnutrition. As noted previously, MAMC may fall before there are changes in serum protein concentrations and thus it provides a relatively early guide to protein depletion. Equations are available for transforming MAMC into total muscle mass but these are not required for routine clinical work.

Both MAC and TSF can be affected by gross fluid overload and thus should be recorded on dialysis patients after a treatment. Figure 1.2 shows the value of anthropometry in a patient with chronic renal

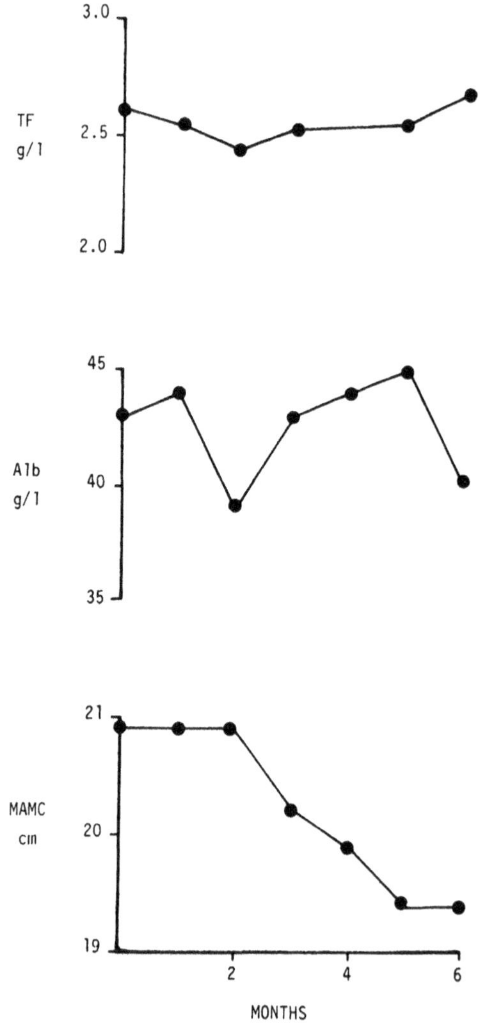

FIGURE 1.2 Serial measurements of serum transferrin (TF), serum albumin (Alb) and mid-arm muscle circumference (MAMC) in a chronic uraemic patient taking a very low nitrogen intake

failure treated with a very low nitrogen intake. The serum proteins stayed within the normal range, but there was a serial fall in MAMC with time implying progressive malnutrition.

NUTRITIONAL REQUIREMENTS

The aim of dietary treatment in chronic renal failure is to provide the patient with sufficient nutrients to prevent depletion without aggravating other aspects of the uraemic state. The nutritional requirements will vary depending on the stage of the illness and the type of treatment being utilized. The question of whether a low protein diet is beneficial before the onset of symptoms will be considered in the next section, p. 22.

General guidelines will be given in this section but it is essential to tailor these to suit the needs of the individual patient. Furthermore, when prescribing any diet it is important to take note of any cultural preferences to improve the chances of compliance.

Pre-dialysis

There is general agreement that protein restriction relieves uraemic symptoms particularly anorexia, nausea and vomiting but there is still controversy over the question, how much should nitrogen intake be restricted in patients with advanced uraemia?

Various studies have utilized a protein consumption from as high as $0.7\,g\,kg^{-1}\,day^{-1}$ to as little as $0.2\,g\,kg^{-1}\,day^{-1}$. Clearly, unless sufficient essential amino acids are given the patient will develop negative nitrogen balance and thus diets of $0.4\,g\,kg^{-1}\,day^{-1}$ or lower have usually been supplemented with essential amino acids or their keto acid analogues. These analogues can be converted *in vivo* to amino acids by transamination and their usage means a further reduction in nitrogen intake.

The proponents of all these regimes report that patients stay in neutral or slightly positive balance but when the more restricted diets are prescribed there is an initial period of nitrogen loss. Unfortunately, very few studies have compared different levels of nitrogen intake. It is, however, clear that essential amino acid or keto acid analogues have no special advantages if the diet contains more than 0.4 g protein kg^{-1} day^{-1}. The lower intakes involve a more complicated regime for the patient and thus this author recommends 0.6 g protein kg^{-1} day^{-1} when protein restriction seems warranted by symptoms. The majority of this protein should be high in biological value. A standard 40 g protein intake should not be prescribed irrespective of patient size. If there is significant proteinuria it is usual to replace losses of more than 2–3 g/day by an equal amount in the diet. It has been claimed that the keto analogue of leucine has special anabolic properties[33], but there has been no clinical comparison with a standard mixed protein intake. The use of keto acid analogues is reported to be associated with a fall in serum parathyroid hormone levels irrespective of total nitrogen or phosphate intake but there are no randomly allocated trials to confirm this finding[34].

It is desirable to reduce phosphate intake in uraemia so that hyperphosphataemia can be more easily controlled. Low protein diets mean a reduction in phosphate but occasionally it is necessary specifically to restrict high phosphate-containing foods such as dairy products.

One of the more difficult problems for the uraemic subject is to consume enough energy. It has recently been shown that the energy expenditure of chronic uraemic patients, both pre-dialysis and on haemodialysis, is the same as normal individuals performing the same activities[35]. It now appears that a minimum of 35 kcal kg^{-1} day^{-1} should be taken if there is not to be a loss of energy stores and possibly increased protein catabolism[36]. A standard British low protein diet requires supplementing with other low protein products, e.g. low protein bread and Caloreen, if this energy requirement is to be met. At the same time the proportion of polyunsaturated to saturated fatty acids in the diet should be increased to unity.

A low protein diet inevitably means a reduction in calcium intake. Care must therefore be taken to ensure that the amount ingested does not fall too low. Supplements such as calcium carbonate, which can also act as a phosphate binder, may be necessary.

If the very low nitrogen intakes are used then there will be a need for additional zinc, B vitamins, vitamin C and sometimes vitamin B_{12} if no animal protein is consumed.

Whether diets giving 0.6 g protein kg^{-1} day^{-1} require supplementing with folic acid is still uncertain. A 70 kg man taking such a regime in the United Kingdom will consume about 120 μg of folic acid per day. There is no longer an official British recommended dietary allowance for normal subjects for this vitamin[37] though in the USA a value of 300–400 μg is advised[20]. Clinical experience suggests that most patients do not develop evidence of folate deficiency even without a supplement and an intake of as little as 100 μg per day has been reported to correct megaloblastic anaemia in non-uraemic individuals. In the United Kingdom tablets of 100 μg, 500 μg and 5 mg can be obtained, but the last is the most widely available. However, if iron is also required then there are numerous combined preparations giving 350 μg per tablet. Pyridoxine (vitamin B_6) has been advised for pre-dialysis patients but the clinical value is uncertain. A standard British low protein diet of 0.6 g/kg usually provides the recommended daily allowance for the other B vitamins.

The sodium and potassium content of the diet will need to be judged on an individual basis. Sodium requires to be restricted in the presence of oedema and/or severe hypertension. Conversely, if the patient is salt wasting sodium supplements are necessary. There is evidence that sodium bicarbonate is of more benefit than sodium chloride as acidosis and nitrogen balance can improve with the former but not the latter[38]. Usually potassium does not cause a problem until the patient requires dialysis but for a minority of patients, specific restrictions of intake may be necessary to help control hyperkalaemia.

TABLE 1.1 Daily dietary allowances for patients with chronic renal failure pre-dialysis

Proteins	0.6 g/kg
Calories	35 kcal/kg
Carbohydrate	40–50% total calories
Fats	30–40% total calories
Polyunsaturated:saturated fatty acids = 1:1	
Calcium	500 mg minimum
Phosphate	< 800 mg
Iron	10 mg
Vitamin supplements	
? Folic acid	1 mg (see text)
? Pyridoxine (B_6)	5 mg
Sodium	to individual requirements

Detailed recommendations are given in Table 1.1. Values expressed per kg body weight relate to ideal or standard weight.

Haemodialysis

There is general agreement that the protein intake of patients receiving regular haemodialysis should be $1.0\,g\,kg^{-1}\,day^{-1}$ or slightly higher. It has been suggested that essential amino acid supplements may further improve the nutritional state but for most subjects this seems unnecessary as long as they can consume the prescribed amount of protein. If all the nitrogen advised is consumed the patient should ingest sufficient calcium. It is, however, important to avoid an excessive phosphate intake so that the need for potentially toxic phosphate-binding drugs can be kept to a minimum. This presents problems since the foods highest in calcium are rich in phosphate. If necessary, calcium supplements such as calcium carbonate should be prescribed to avoid excess phosphate consumption.

Calorie and lipid requirements are the same as for pre-dialysis patients. Sodium intake has to be restricted by the majority of patients to help control fluid overload and hypertension. Potassium intake usually needs to be controlled though a small minority of patients may be allowed a free intake to prevent hypokalaemia. Fluid intake requires restriction in the vast majority of cases. It has become traditional to prescribe supplementary vitamins B and C, though recently it has been claimed that this is not necessary for many patients[22]. In view of their low cost and safety, however, it is probably wiser to continue these drugs for the time being. In the United Kingdom the recent restriction on National Health Service prescribing has limited the availability of multi-vitamin preparations. Thus the full recommendations can only be met if the patient takes 4 tablets a day namely, vitamin B compound strong giving thiamine 5 mg and some other B vitamins, pyridoxine 10 mg, ascorbic acid 50 mg and folic acid 5 mg. The last drug is in excess of requirements but is apparently harmless. Larger doses of ascorbic acid, e.g. 500 mg/day, may actually be deleterious as they have been associated with raised serum oxalate levels. Iron should be prescribed if iron deficiency occurs. Ferrous sulphate is the most suitable preparation (detailed recommendations are given in Table 1.2).

Haemofiltration or haemodiafiltration involves the use of much more permeable membranes and a considerably greater flux of plasma water during treatment than with haemodialysis. No firm data are yet available but it is likely that losses of all water-soluble vitamins will be much greater and therefore supplements should be prescribed as a routine.

TABLE 1.2 Daily dietary allowances for patients receiving regular haemodialysis

Protein	1.0–1.2 g/kg
Calories	35 kcal/kg
Carbohydrates	40% total calories
Fats	30–40% total calories
Polyunsaturated:saturated fatty acids = 1:1	
Calcium	1000 mg minimum
Phosphate	<1000 mg if possible
Iron	As necessary
Vitamin supplements	
B_1	2 mg
B_6	10 mg
C	50 mg
Folic acid	1 mg
Sodium	To individual requirement
Potassium	Majority of patients require a restriction
Fluid	To suit individual, may be as little as 500 ml

Peritoneal dialysis

Patients receiving any form of peritoneal dialysis are subject to considerable losses of protein. Thus their protein intake needs to be higher than for patients receiving haemodialysis. At least 1.3 g kg^{-1} day^{-1} is recommended[39]. Similar requirements for calcium and phosphate apply as for haemodialysis.

CAPD involves the infusion of large amounts of dextrose and it is thus not surprising that this has been calculated to contribute 300–800 kcal/day depending on the concentration used[13]. There is evidence that CAPD patients tend to suppress their carbohydrate intake in proportion to the dialysate dextrose absorbed. Patients are advised to avoid concentrated carbohydrate sources in the diet.

Sodium and water intake needs to be restricted as for haemodialysis but in general CAPD patients are able to have a more liberal potassium content in the diet.

Water-soluble vitamins are lost in the dialysis procedure and plasma levels may fall in patients treated by CAPD[40]. As with haemodialysis, occasional cases of folic acid deficiency have been reported. Though the clinical value is still uncertain at present it would seem wise to supplement the diet with vitamins B_1, B_6, C and folic acid.

Many patients on CAPD tend to reduce their food intake with time[13]. Their decreased appetite is caused partly by abdominal distension from CAPD fluid and partly by peritoneal absorption of dextrose. Dietary compliance should thus be assessed regularly (Table 1.3). Constipation exacerbated by the fluid restriction is a problem experienced by many patients. A high fibre diet, of bran or unrefined cereals, is recommended.

TABLE 1.3 Daily dietary allowances for patients receiving CAPD

Protein	1.3–1.5 g/kg
Calories	35 kcal/kg. NB Glucose absorption variable from dialysate
Carbohydrate	40% total calories
Fat	30–40% total calories
Polyunsaturated:saturated fatty acids = 1:1	
Calcium	1000 mg minimum
Phosphate	<1000 mg if possible
Vitamin supplements	
B_1	2 mg
B_6	5 mg
C	50 mg
Folic acid	1 mg
Potassium	Majority of patients no restriction necessary

NB Restrict use of bags with increased dextrose by limiting fluid intake

Children

In addition to the other problems already noted, uraemic malnutrition in children also contributes to growth retardation. The severity of this phenomenon depends partly on the age of the child at the onset of uraemia. Pre-pubertal children are more severely affected and infants suffer most of all. A detailed consideration of the nutritional requirements of uraemic children is to be found in Chapter 2.

Intercurrent problems

The recommended regimes noted above are adequate to keep most patients in reasonable health. Despite the best efforts, nutritional status will deteriorate if either there are increased requirements due to catabolism from illness or food intake becomes inadequate. Unfortunately, it is all too easy to forget the patient is not having enough nutrients or to assume that any such problem will be short lived; serious undernutrition may occur before remedial action is taken. Even patients who are not otherwise ill may ingest inadequate quantities of food. Surveys have shown that most dialysis patients consume their recommended protein allowance but many take considerably fewer calories than prescribed. It is therefore essential that supplementary feeding should be provided early if there is any evidence that the patient's nutritional requirements are not being met.

The simplest type of supplement is in the form of powder, protein or carbohydrate, which can be mixed into the food and thus avoid additional fluid intake. Concentrated carbohydrate is available in liquid form but does not contain monosaccharides which would make it too sweet. Various formulations of oral feeds are also available to be made up as a water-based drink or milkshake depending on the patient's preference. If these cannot be easily tolerated then continuous nasogastric feeding via a fine bore tube should be tried. The mixtures used can be formulated to meet individual requirements and contain all necessary minerals, metals and vitamins. Sometimes overnight feeding may prove sufficient. This technique is usually well tolerated by patients and ensures a minimum intake of up to 40 g of protein and 1000 calories in 1000 ml plus anything the individual consumes by mouth. Though this is an additional fluid load to the body, in our experience haemodialysis three times a week or CAPD can still control fluid balance. Only when the gastrointestinal tract cannot be used should full parenteral feeding be considered. In this eventuality, continuous haemofiltration will easily remove the quantities of fluid involved.

It is, however, possible to supplement diets for haemodialysis patients by infusing with amino acids and carbohydrates during the dialysis procedure. This allows the fluid load to be removed immediately and although there is a slight increased loss of amino acids in the dialysate the majority are retained in the body. If carbohydrate is infused there may be reactive hypoglycaemia but a carbohydrate meal at the end of dialysis prevents this phenomenon. If gross hypoalbuminaemia is present then intravenous protein may be required.

When anorexia seems to be the main problem despite good control of uraemia, zinc ingestion has been reported to be beneficial and is certainly harmless when given for just a few weeks. Zinc sulphate 220 mg twice a week seems to be an adequate dose.

INFLUENCE OF DIET ON PROGRESSIVE RENAL FAILURE

There is now general agreement that once a certain degree of chronic renal failure has occurred renal function continues to deteriorate even when the original cause is no longer operational. Thus patients with uraemia due to malignant hypertension or obstructive uropathy may still progress to end-stage renal failure despite adequate treatment. It has been suggested that the renal damage becomes self-propagating by mechanisms that are not specific for the original cause and are operational in any patient with progressive uraemia. Currently, there are three theories to explain this process. Firstly, further damage is thought to be due to haemodynamic disturbances in the remaining glomeruli[41]. Single nephron glomerular filtration increases and as a consequence macromolecules accumulate in the mesangium with subsequent progressive glomerulosclerosis. The exact sequence of events is still uncertain but intraglomerular hypertension appears to play a key role and this in turn is mediated by the balance between afferent and efferent arteriolar resistance. The second hypothesis is that deposition of calcium phosphate (in renal tissue) and possibly urate and oxalate as well, leads to an inflammatory and fibrotic response. Finally, it has been suggested that plasma lipids, in particular lipoproteins, could contribute to glomerular pathology. These proposed mechanisms are not mutually exclusive and all could be altered by dietary manipulation. Thus there is considerable interest in the potential role of the diet in slowing or halting progressive renal failure.

Experimental

There are two main models of progressive uraemia in animals, namely subtotal or five-sixths nephrectomy and nephrotoxic nephritis both using the rat. In both examples animals fed a low protein diet live longer, have less proteinuria and a low serum creatinine. This beneficial effect of a low nitrogen intake has been shown repeatedly over many years[42,43]. More recently, it has been suggested that a low phosphate intake may have a protective role in experimental uraemia. Unfortunately, the original reports failed to note that the animals also had reduced consumption of other nutrients, particularly protein. However, it is now claimed that reduction of phosphate absorption alone protects experimental animals from progressive renal failure[44]. There have been only a few studies looking at the influence of lipids, but there is some evidence that polyunsaturated fatty acids may be beneficial in animal models of chronic uraemia[45].

Clinical

In view of the dramatic effects of protein restriction in experimental animals it is not surprising that there have been a considerable number of studies trying varying degrees of nitrogen intake reduction in patients with chronic renal failure. Virtually all published work to date has claimed that low protein diets are beneficial in man and there is a body of opinion advocating the widespread use of such regimes in asymptomatic individuals[46]. Unfortunately, most of the reports suffer from a number of deficiencies[47].

Implicit in the use of a low protein diet is the assumption that without treatment, renal function will inevitably deteriorate. This is not necessarily true. Figure 1.3 shows the course of one patient with chronic renal failure followed for 17 years. Renal function remained stable even though protein intake was normal at $1.2\,g\,kg^{-1}\,day^{-1}$. Several published studies have shown that a considerable number of patients with different renal conditions have stable function for several years. Despite this well-known fact, some of the reports claiming benefit from a low protein diet have followed patients for only a few months and/or did not establish that patients had progressive renal impairment before starting treatment; thus any benefit claimed could have been due to the variable natural history. Important prognostic factors in human uraemia include age, sex, type of disease, presence of hypertension, degree of proteinuria and degree of renal impairment when first seen. To date no study has taken all these influences into account.

The next difficulty in assessing dietary treatment is the reliability of different methods of measuring progression. Most reports have looked at the reciprocal creatinine plot before and after starting on a diet. This method is, however, invalid since after reduction of protein intake there is an alteration in creatinine metabolism which is not related to

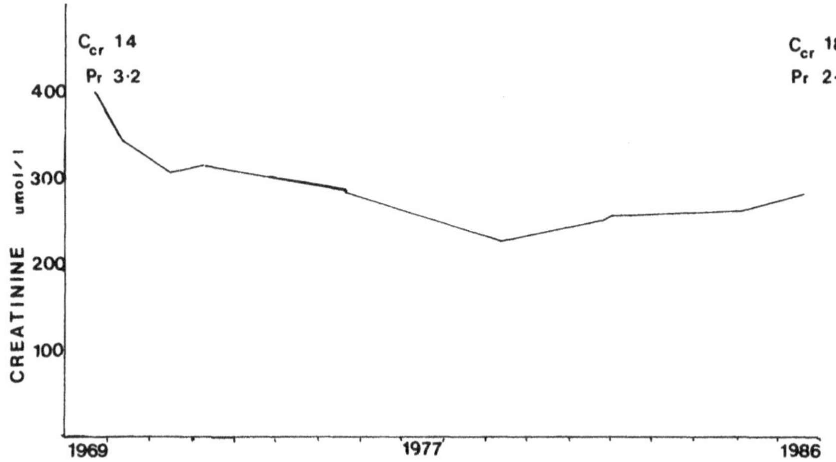

FIGURE 1.3 Plasma creatinine measurements during 17-year follow-up in a patient with chronic renal failure. C_{cr} = creatinine clearance in ml/min; Pr = 24-hour urinary protein in grams

changes in renal function[48]. It is due partly to reduced meat consumption, sometimes a loss of muscle mass and also an alteration in endogenous metabolism. Although it has been suggested that 3–4 months are required to reach a new steady state[49], all studies claiming benefit have looked at the reciprocal creatinine from the time of starting the diet and thus the results are not a valid assessment of renal function. A few reports have provided information on creatinine clearance but this is also known to be an inaccurate marker of renal function, particularly in advanced uraemia[50]. To date, there are no published data on inulin or isotopic clearances in relation to slowing the progression of renal failure with the exception of studies on the control of hypertension in diabetics.

So far only one report has appeared in which the patients were randomly allocated to treatment or control groups and then prospectively followed[51]. In the majority of the other studies the patients acted as their own controls. The remainder of published work in this field has included data on individuals who were not receiving a diet but none of these constituted appropriate controls. The only randomly allocated study did claim benefit from a low protein diet but the method of assessment used changes in serum creatinine and thus some doubt has been cast on the conclusions.

Since the majority of reports have used patients as their own controls, it is important to be sure there is no placebo effect. It is now clear that there is undoubtedly a clinic effect[52]. The natural consequence of starting a diet is that patients are reviewed more often than before. It has recently been shown that more frequent follow-up alone produces a slowing in the rate of progression of renal failure, probably due to better control of blood pressure.

Another difficulty in deciding whether low protein regimes are beneficial is that there has been a considerable variation in nitrogen intake in different reports. The very low protein diets have usually been supplemented by essential amino acids and/or keto acid analogues. To date, there has been no comparison of the relative merits of the different regimes.

The major concern when prescribing any low nitrogen diet is to prevent the patient from developing malnutrition. Papers claiming benefit from such regimes have provided information on weight and serum proteins, but rarely any anthropometric data. However, one study of a very low protein essential amino acid–keto acid diet did provide evidence that considerable loss of muscle mass could occur[53]. Whether less restricted diets also have a nutritional price remains uncertain.

Thus the case for using low protein diets to slow the progression of renal failure has not yet been proved in man. Several large multicentre controlled trials are currently in progress in an attempt to resolve this question.

All human diets low in protein also inevitably restrict phosphorus. There is one report of an uncontrolled study claiming that a very low phosphate, low nitrogen intake is more beneficial than a low nitrogen diet alone, but further data are necessary[53]. So far, there is no information on the value of altering lipids in the diet on the progression of human chronic renal failure.

ASSESSMENT OF DIETARY COMPLIANCE

It is important to assess the patient's compliance with any prescribed diet since deviations may produce clinically serious results. A number of techniques are available and the appropriate ones should be used in combination depending on the stage of the illness.

Dietary history

The only exact way of assessing the quantity and quality of food that a patient consumes is to analyse weighed aliquots of everything eaten. This clearly requires the facilities of a full metabolic ward. For outpatients weighing all meal portions for several days each month is fairly reliable but tedious. The patient is asked to weigh and record on specially prepared sheets each item of food consumed over a 4-day period. On return to the clinic a dietitian should then interview the patient to check the facts and provide advice for any queries or difficulties. Usually the spouse or other close relative is also seen to corroborate the record. The sheets are then converted into nutritional equivalents using tables of the composition of foods. This process has now been greatly simplified as programs containing all the tables are available for microcomputers. The dietitian has to enter the common name of each item and its quantity. When all items have been listed the computer will print out a complete record of the average daily intake of proteins, carbohydrates, fats, metals, vitamins, etc. and thus compliance can be rapidly assessed and corrective action taken well before the next scheduled visit. This method of assessment has been shown to be reliable when performed by an experienced dietitian and compares well with more formal measurements. A dietary history can be used at any stage of the treatment of chronic renal failure but should cover dialysis and non-dialysis days if the patient is receiving haemodialysis.

Urea/creatinine ratio

Once a protein-restricted diet is started the blood urea will be proportionately lower for the same plasma creatinine. Thus the ratio gives a rough idea of the rate of urea formation. Higher values either mean dietary indiscretion or increased catabolism[54]. Any factor which independently alters creatinine concentration will tend to invalidate the ratio. Thus patients with reduced muscle mass, e.g. children, small women and those with wasting, will have a relatively lower plasma creatinine for the same level of renal function. Furthermore, as noted previously, there is evidence that with very low protein intakes there may be an initial fall in creatinine independent of changes in glomerular filtration rate. Thus the actual value of the ratio will vary from patient to patient, but if an individual has previously been in a steady state an alteration in the ratio may prove a useful marker of potential nutritional problems. This technique is not applicable for assessing dietary compliance of dialysis patients.

Urea nitrogen appearance

Urea is the major nitrogenous product of protein, particularly in uraemic patients, and urinary urea excretion appears to vary directly with protein intake. Urea nitrogen appearance (UNA) is defined as the sum of urinary urea nitrogen plus the change in body urea nitrogen[54]. It represents net but not total urea production as some urea is recycled via the gut to ammonia which is then reabsorbed and converted back to urea in the liver.

UNA is calculated as follows:

$$\text{UNA (gN/day)} = \text{Urinary urea N (g/day)} + [(\text{Blood urea nitrogen}_f - \text{Blood urea nitrogen}_i) \times 0.6 \times \text{Body weight}_i] + [(\text{Body weight}_f - \text{Body weight}_i) \times \text{Blood urea nitrogen}_f]$$

where i and f represent initial and final values over the period of measurement, usually 1–3 days. Blood urea nitrogen is measured in g/litre, body weight in kilograms and 0.6 represents an estimate of the total body water content of body weight. The latter will require correction in subjects who are oedematous, obese, wasted or very young. Changes in body weight are assumed to be due to alterations in body water. Table 1.4 provides appropriate conversions of urea concentrations obtained as millimole/litre. For outpatients the 24-hour urinary urea excretion alone is a close approximation to UNA unless the blood urea and/or body weight has changed markedly. UNA underestimates true nitrogen intake when the patient is in nitrogen balance since a proportion is excreted as non-urea nitrogen in the urine and faeces. Recently it has been shown that non-urea nitrogen is related to weight and does not vary with different protein intakes[55]. Thus a true assessment of nitrogen excretion requires a correction

TABLE 1.4 Urea Nitrogen appearance. Conversion of SI units to grams

1 gram molecular weight of urea = 60 grams = 1 mole
Nitrogen content of 1 mol of urea = 28 grams

To convert urea as mmol/l to urea N as g/l:
Multiply by 28 and divide by 1000

Thus urinary urea N g/day =

$$\frac{\text{Urinary urea mmol/l} \times \text{24 hour urine vol (l)} \times 28}{1000}$$

$$\text{Blood urea nitrogen g/l} = \frac{\text{Blood urea mmol/l} \times 28}{1000}$$

factor as follows:

$$\text{Total nitrogen excretion g/day} = \text{UNA} + 31\ \text{mg kg}^{-1}\ \text{day}^{-1}.$$

This estimate correlates well with values obtained by direct measurement in a metabolic ward, although there is a possible error of up to 2 g of nitrogen per day for a large individual (>80 kg) with the use of this correction factor. Despite this, corrected UNA provides a valuable estimate of dietary compliance of patients in approximately neutral nitrogen balance. If a dietary history is taken at the same time, nitrogen balance can be estimated.

Urea kinetics

The previous technique requires adjustment before it can be used for patients receiving haemodialysis. The modified method calculates net urea generation and is commonly called urea kinetics[56]. The necessary information required is as follows:

Residual renal urea clearance
Dialyser urea clearance at patient's blood flow
Length of time of dialysis
Pre- and post-dialysis blood urea concentrations
Patient's weight

Usually pre- and post-urea concentrations are obtained for two consecutive dialyses together with a pre-value before the third. The equations used in the calculations estimate the total urea removed during this period and also urea generation. The volume of distribution of urea (total body water) is usually derived by an iterative technique. From the urea generation the protein catabolic rate can be calculated and this should equal protein intake if the patient is in neutral balance. Discrepancies can be checked with the dietary history as before and thus increased catabolism or indiscretion detected. The equations used in this method of assessment are complex and require a programmable calculator or microcomputer to solve. However nomograms have been published to assist clinicians in the use of urea kinetics[57].

If the protein catabolic rate is known this technique can also be used to assess the dialysis requirements of an individual patient.

Peritoneal dialysis

Since peritoneal dialysis inevitably means losses of protein as well as urea and other nitrogenous metabolites, there is no simple way of assessing nitrogen balance and thus dietary compliance. Direct measurement of all nitrogen losses in the dialysate would be necessary for any degree of accuracy. However, if the patient's serum albumin is normal it can be assumed the patient is consuming sufficient protein. In the presence of hypoalbuminaemia a dietary history together with a search for excessive losses and/or increased catabolism will be required to determine the cause of the problem.

Calorie intake

Methods of assessing dietary compliance using urea are valuable for determining protein intake. Unfortunately, apart from dietary history, there is no independent method for checking calorie consumption. In the long term, changes in skinfold thickness (body fat) will be of most value.

FUTURE TRENDS

If dietary change can alter the progression of chronic renal disease in man, then much greater attention will have to be directed to nutrition by nephrologists in the future. Among dietary possibilities of unproven value, the ingestion of fish oil is currently attracting most attention. Fish oil contains eicosapentaenoic acid (EPA) which acts as an analogue for arachidonic acid. As a consequence, different prostaglandins, thromboxanes and leukotrienes are produced by the cyclo-oxygenase and lipoxygenase pathways respectively. These alternative derivatives have somewhat different actions to those produced from arachidonic acid. Short-term studies in man using EPA as a dietary supplement have shown alterations in blood polymorph and monocyte function in normal subjects[58] and improved plasma lipids together with decreased platelet aggregability in haemodialysis patients[59]. The long-term safety of such a regime is unknown but fish oil might prove beneficial in slowing the progression of renal failure as there is some evidence that the balance between prostaglandins and thromboxane may contribute to the loss of function in an experimental model.

ACKNOWLEDGEMENTS

I am grateful to Miss Judyth Meadows, Chief Dietitian, Cardiff Royal Infirmary, for many helpful discussions and to Miss Tracey Richards, Renal Pharmacist, Cardiff Royal Infirmary, for advice on the availability of vitamin supplements. Miss Rita Sultana kindly typed the manuscript.

References

1. Guarnieri, G., Faccini, L., Lipartiti, T., Ranieri, F., Spangaro, F., Guintini, D., Toigo, G., Dardi, F., Berquier-Vidali, F. and Raimondi, A. (1980). Simple methods for nutritional assessment in hemodialyzed patients. *Am. J. Clin. Nutr.*, **33,** 1598–607
2. Thunberg, B. J., Swamy, A. P. and Cestero, R. V. M. (1981). Cross sectional and longitudinal nutritional measurements in maintenance hemodialysis patients. *Am. J. Clin. Nutr.*, **34,** 2005–12
3. Coles, G. A. (1972). Body composition in chronic renal failure. *Q. J. Med.*, **41,** 25–47
4. Mitch, W. E. and Wilcox, C. S. (1982). Disorders of body fluids, sodium and potassium in chronic renal failure. *Am. J. Med.*, **72,** 536–50
5. Kopple, J. D. (1978). Abnormal amino acid and protein metabolism in uremia. *Kidney Int.*, **14,** 340–8
6. Coles, G. A., Peters, D. K. and Jones, J. H. (1970). Albumin metabolism in chronic renal failure. *Clin. Sci.*, **39,** 423–35
7. Bianchi, R., Mariani, G., Toni, M. G. and Carmassi, F. (1978). The metabolism of human serum albumin in renal failure on conservative and dialysis therapy. *Am. J. Clin. Nutr.*, **31,** 1615–26
8. Kayser, G. A. and Schoenfeld, P. Y. (1984). Albumin homeostasis in patients undergoing continuous ambulatory peritoneal dialysis. *Kidney Int.*, **25,** 107–14
9. Guarnieri, G., Toigo, G., Situlin, R., Faccini, L., Coli, U., Landini, S., Bazzato, G., Dardi, F. and Campanacci, L. (1983). Muscle biopsy studies in chronically uraemic patients: evidence for malnutrition. *Kidney Int.*, **24,** Suppl 16, S187–93
10. Li, J. B. and Wassner, S. J. (1986). Protein synthesis and degradation in skeletal muscle of chronically uremic rats. *Kidney Int.*, **29,** 1136–43
11. Fürst, P., Alvestrand, A. and Bergström, J. (1980). Effects of nutrition and catabolic stress on intracellular amino acid pools in uremia. *Am. J. Clin. Nutr.*, **33,** 1387–95

12. Alvestrand, A. and Bergström, J. (1984). Nutritional management. In Suki, W. N. and Massry, S. G. (eds.) *Therapy of Renal Diseases and Related Disorders*. pp. 459–80. (Boston: Martinus Nijhoff)
13. Lindholm, B. and Bergström, J. (1986). Nutritional aspects of CAPD. In Gokal, R. (ed.) *Continuous Ambulatory Peritoneal Dialysis*. pp. 228–64 (Edinburgh: Churchill Livingstone)
14. Ibels, L. S., Reardon, M. F. and Nestel, P. J. (1976). Plasma post-heparin lipolytic activity and triglyceride clearance in uremic and hemodialysis patients and renal allograft recipients. *J. Lab. Clin. Med.*, **87**, 648–58
15. Ramos, J. M., Heaton, A., McGurk, J. G., Ward, M. K. and Kerr, D. N. S. (1983). Sequential changes in serum lipids and their subfractions in patients receiving continuous ambulatory peritoneal dialysis. *Nephron*, **35**, 20–3
16. Guarnieri, G. F., Ranieri, F., Toigo, G., Vasile, A., Ciman, M., Rizzoli, V., Moracchiello, M. and Campanacci, L. (1980). Lipid lowering effect of carnitine in chronically uremic patients treated with maintenance hemodialysis. *Am. J. Clin. Nutr.*, **33**, 1489–92
17. Wanner, C., Forstner-Wanner, S., Schaeffer, G., Schollmeyer, P. and Horl, W. H. (1986). Serum free carnitine, carnitine esters and lipids in patients on peritoneal dialysis and hemodialysis. *Am. J. Nephrol.*, **6**, 206–11
18. Sanfelippo, N. L., Swenson, R. S. and Reaven, G. M. (1977). Reduction of plasma triglycerides by diet in subjects with chronic renal failure. *Kidney Int.*, **11**, 54–61
19. Gokal, R. S., Mann, J. I., Oliver, D. O., Ledingham, J. G. G. and Carter, R. D. (1978). Treatment of hyperlipidaemia in patients on chronic haemodialysis. *Br. Med. J.*, **1**, 82–3
20. Kopple, J. D. and Swendseid, M. E. (1975). Vitamin nutrition in patients undergoing maintenance hemodialysis. *Kidney Int.*, **7**, Suppl. 2, S79–84
21. Kopple, J. D., Mercurio, K., Blumenkrantz, M. J., Jones, M. R., Tallos, J., Roberts, C., Card, B., Saltzmann, R., Casciato, D. A. and Swendseid, M. E. (1981). Daily requirement for pyridoxine supplements in chronic renal failure. *Kidney Int.*, **19**, 694–704
22. Ramirez, G., Chen, M., Boyce, H. W., Fuller, S. M., Ganguly, R., Brueggemeyer, C. D. and Butcher, D. E. (1986). Longitudinal follow-up of chronic hemodialysis patients without vitamin supplementation. *Kidney Int.*, **30**, 99–106
23. Alfrey, A. C. and Smythe, W. R. (1986). Trace metals and regular dialysis. In Drukker, W., Parsons, F. M. and Maher, J. F. (eds.) *Replacement of Renal Function by Dialysis*. pp. 804–10. (Dordrecht: Martinus Nijhoff)
24. Halder, M. and Halder, S. Q. (1984). Assessment of protein-calorie malnutrition. *Clin. Chem.*, **30**, 1286–99
25. Hobbs, C. L., Murray, T. G. and Mullen, J. L. (1979). Implications of malnutrition in chronic renal hemodialysis patients. *J. Parent. Ent. Nutr.*, **3**, 27
26. Young, G. A., Young, J. B., Young, S. M., Hobson, S. M., Hildreth, B., Brownjohn, A. M. and Parsons, F. M. (1986). Nutrition and delayed hypersensitivity during continuous ambulatory peritoneal dialysis in relation to peritonitis. *Nephron*, **43**, 177–86
27. Degoulet, P., Reach, I., Aime, F., Rioux, P., Jacobs, C. and Legrain, M. (1980). Risk factors in chronic haemodialysis. *Proc. Eur. Dial. Transplant Assoc.*, **17**, 149–53
28. Wolfson, W., Strong, C. J., Minturn, D., Gray, D. K. and Kopple, J. D. (1984). Nutritional status and lymphocyte function in maintenance hemodialysis patients. *Am. J. Clin. Nutr.*, **39**, 547–55

29. Berkelhammer, C. H., Leiter, L. A., Jeejeebhoy, K. N., Detsky, A. S., Oreopoulos, D. G., Uldall, P. R. and Baker, J. P. (1985). Skeletal muscle function in chronic renal failure: an index of nutritional status. *Am. J. Clin. Nutr.*, **42,** 845–54
30. Truswell, A. S. (1985). Measuring nutrition. *Br. Med. J.*, **29,** 1258–62
31. Blumenkrantz, M. J., Kopple, J. D., Gutman, R. A., Chan, Y. K., Barbour, G. L., Roberts, C., Shen, F. H., Gandhi, V. C., Tucker, C. T., Curtis, F. K. and Coburn, J. W. (1980). Methods for assessing nutritional status of patients with renal failure. *Am. J. Clin. Nutr.*, **33,** 1567–85
32. Harvey, K. B., Blumenkrantz, M. J., Levine, S. E. and Blackburn, G. L. (1980). Nutritional assessment and treatment of chronic renal failure. *Am. J. Clin. Nutr.*, **33,** 1586–97
33. Mitch, W. E. (1980). Metabolism and metabolic effects of ketoacids. *Am. J. Clin. Nutr.*, **33,** 1642–8
34. Lindenau, K., Kokot, F. and Frohling, P. T. (1986). Suppression of parathyroid hormone by therapy with a mixture of keto analogues of amino acids in hemodialysis patients. *Nephron*, **43,** 84–6
35. Monteon, F. J., Laidlaw, S. A., Shaib, J. K. and Kopple, J. D. (1986). Energy expenditure in patients with chronic renal failure. *Kidney Int.*, **30,** 741–7
36. Kopple, J. D., Monteon, F. J. and Shaib, J. K. (1986). Effect of energy intake on nitrogen metabolism in nondialyzed patients with chronic renal failure. *Kidney Int.*, **29,** 734–42
37. Committee on medical aspects of food policy (1979). Recommended daily amounts of food energy and nutrients for groups of people in the United Kingdom. *DHSS Report on health and social subjects*, **15**
38. Papadoyannakis, N. J., Stefanidis, C. J. and McGeown, M. (1984). The effect of the correction of metabolic acidosis on nitrogen and potassium balance of patients with chronic renal failure. *Am. J. Clin. Nutr.*, **40,** 623–7
39. Blumenkrantz, M. J., Kopple, J. D., Moran, J. K. and Coburn, J. W. (1982). Metabolic balance studies and dietary protein requirements in patients undergoing continuous ambulatory peritoneal dialysis. *Kidney Int.*, **21,** 849–61
40. Blumberg, A., Hanck, A. and Sander, G. (1983). Vitamin nutrition in patients on continuous ambulatory peritoneal dialysis (CAPD). *Clin. Neph.*, **20,** 244–50
41. Brenner, B. M. (1985). Nephron adaptation to renal injury or ablation. *Am. J. Physiol.*, **249,** F324–37
42. Farr, L. E. and Smadel, J. E. (1940). The effect of dietary protein on the course of nephrotoxic nephritis in rats. *Am. J. Pathol.*, **16,** 615–27
43. Klahr, S., Buekert, J. and Purkerson, M. L. (1983). Role of dietary factors in the progression of chronic renal disease. *Kidney Int.*, **24,** 579–87
44. Lumlertgul, D., Burke, T. J., Gillum, D. M., Alfrey, A. C., Harris, D. C., Hammond, D. S. and Schrier, R. W. (1986). Phosphate depletion arrests progression of chronic renal failure independent of protein intake. *Kidney Int.*, **29,** 658–66
45. Barcelli, U. and Pollak, V. E. (1985). Is there a role for polyunsaturated fatty acids in the prevention of renal disease and renal failure? *Nephron*, **41,** 209–12
46. Giovanetti, S. (1985). Dietary treatment of chronic renal failure: why is it not used more frequently? *Nephron*, **40,** 1–12
47. El Nahas, A. M. and Coles, G. A. (1986). Dietary treatment of chronic renal failure: ten unanswered questions. *Lancet*, **1,** 597–600

48. Lucas, P. A., Meadows, J. H., Roberts, D. E. and Coles, G. A. (1986). The risks and benefits of a low protein–essential amino acid–keto acid diet. *Kidney Int.*, **29,** 995–1003
49. Mitch, W. E. (1984). The influence of the diet on the progression of renal insufficiency. *Ann. Rev. Med.*, **35,** 249–64
50. Shemesh, O., Golbetz, H., Kriss, J.P. and Myers, B. D. (1985). Limitations of creatinine as a filtration marker in glomerulopathic patients. *Kidney Int.*, **28,** 830–8
51. Rosman, J. B., Ter Wee, P. M., Meijer, S., Piers-Becht, T. P. M., Sluiter, W. M. and Donker, A. J. M. (1984). Prospective randomised trial of early dietary protein restriction in chronic renal failure. *Lancet,* **1,** 1291–6
52. Bergström, J., Alvestrand, A., Bucht, H. and Gutierrez, A. (1986). Progression of chronic renal failure in man is retarded with more frequent clinical follow-ups and better blood pressure control. *Clin. Neph.*, **25,** 1–6
53. Barsotti, G., Giannoni, A., Morelli, E., Lazzeri, M., Vlamis, I., Baldi, R. and Giovanetti, S. (1984). The decline of renal function slowed by very low phosphorus intake in chronic renal patients following a low nitrogen diet. *Clin. Neph.*, **21,** 54–9
54. Kopple, J. D., Roberts, C. E., Grodstein, G. P., Shah, G. M., Winer, R. L., Davidson, W. D., Henry, D. A. and Franklin, S. S. (1982). Low protein diets and the nondialyzed uremic patient. In Avram, N. M. (ed.) *Prevention of Kidney Disease and Long Term Survival.* pp. 3–22. (New York: Plenum)
55. Maroni, B. J., Steinman, T. I. and Mitch, W. E. (1985). A method for estimating nitrogen intake of patients with chronic renal failure. *Kidney Int.*, **27,** 58–65
56. Sargent, J., Gotch, F., Borek, M., Piercy, L., Spinozzi, N., Schoenfield, P. and Humphreys, M. (1978). Urea kinetics: a guide to nutritional management of renal failure. *Am. J. Clin. Nutr.*, **31,** 1696–702
57. Gotch, F. A. (1986). Urea kinetic modelling to guide hemodialysis therapy in adults. In Nissenson, A. R. and Fine, R. N. (eds.) *Dialysis Therapy.* pp. 66–9. (Philadelphia: Hanley and Belfus, Inc.)
58. Lee, T. H., Hoover, R. L., Williams, J. D., Sperling, R. I., Ravalese, J., Spur, B. W., Robinson, D. R., Corey, E. J., Lewis, R. A. and Austen, K. F. (1985). Effect of dietary enrichment with eicosapentaenoic and docosahexaenoic acids on *in vitro* neutrophil and monocyte leukotriene generation and neutrophil function. *N. Engl. J. Med.*, **312,** 1217–24
59. Rylance, P. B., Gordge, M. P., Saynor, R., Parsons, V. and Weston, M. J. (1986). Fish oil modifies lipids and reduces platelet aggregability in haemodialysis patients. *Nephron,* **43,** 196–202

2

MANAGEMENT OF CHILDREN WITH CHRONIC RENAL FAILURE

A. V. MURPHY

INTRODUCTION

In California in 1967 children were first accepted on to long-term haemodialysis paediatric programmes[1,2]. The experience from these centres led to other paediatric dialysis programmes being set up elsewhere in America, Canada and Europe. In 1972 facilities became available at the Royal Hospital for Sick Children, Glasgow. Since that time there have been radical changes in the management, from the conservative treatment of potentially fatal disease to the fairly aggressive therapy of even small infants with renal failure.

In chronic renal failure of childhood, three main phases can be discerned; the length of time in each phase corresponds to the underlying disease and varies from months to many years. In phase 1, more than 50% of normal renal function is preserved and the child is generally asymptomatic. He may present, however, with secondary enuresis from polyuria and a decrease in growth velocity may be noted[3]. It is important in this stage that any reversible factors should be looked for and treated. Hypertension diagnosed and managed effectively may lessen the rate of deterioration in renal function and treatment of anaemia and failure to thrive can improve the quality of life.

In phase 2 renal function is less than 50% of normal. Bone pain from renal osteodystrophy may occur and systemic acidosis may contribute to a further reduction in growth as the renal function falls to 10% of normal. Symptoms of itch, lethargy and anorexia become progressive. Dietary measures are important. A polydipsic phase of renal failure can be replaced quite suddenly by oliguria and the child may present as an emergency with acute pulmonary oedema. When renal function deteriorates to less than 10% of normal in phase 3, life is, in general, not supported without artificial means.

COMPLICATIONS OF RENAL FAILURE

Hypertension

Children with chronic renal failure may have hypertension. This may be caused by the primary disease process itself or be secondary to the sodium and water overload associated with advanced renal failure. Early and effective control of hypertension is mandatory. Children tolerate relatively large doses of β-blocking drugs. Atenolol (1–2 mg kg^{-1} day^{-1}) is the drug of first choice. The vasodilator hydralazine (1–8 mg kg^{-1} day^{-1}) can be added if required. The addition of prazosin (0.05–0.4 mg kg^{-1} day^{-1}) often controls a particularly resistant blood pressure. Side-effects on these three drugs are uncommon, although there may be complaints of headache with hydralazine. Children who have their hypertension managed early and effectively can show a progressive rise in the glomerular filtration rate which can remain static for many years thereafter.

The child with chronic renal failure disease may present with acute hypertensive encephalopathy – drowsiness, convulsions and hallucinations. Intravenous antihypertensive therapy is usually necessary and the combined α and β blocking drug, labetalol, infused at 1–3 mg kg^{-1} h^{-1} i.v. can produce effective control. If not, then the vasodilator sodium nitroprusside 0.5–0.8 μg kg^{-1} min^{-1} i.v. may be useful. When sodium and water overload is present the effect of treatment with intravenous diuretics in high dosage may be assessed, but fluid restriction and preparation for dialysis are generally indicated.

Obstructive uropathy

Children with obstructive uropathy require detailed investigation of their renal tracts with regular combined supervision from the paediatric urologist and nephrologist. Obstructive lesions occur most commonly in children with neurogenic bladder or as a result of spina bifida or spinal deformities. If there is dysynergia of the detrusor sphincter with vesicoureteric reflux, loss of functioning renal tissue can occur over a short time. Figures 2.1 and 2.2 show the micturating cysto-urethrogram and DMSA scan in a 2-year-old child with a severely dysplastic left kidney contributing only 8% of overall function; 1 year previously renal ultrasound demonstrated a normal left kidney.

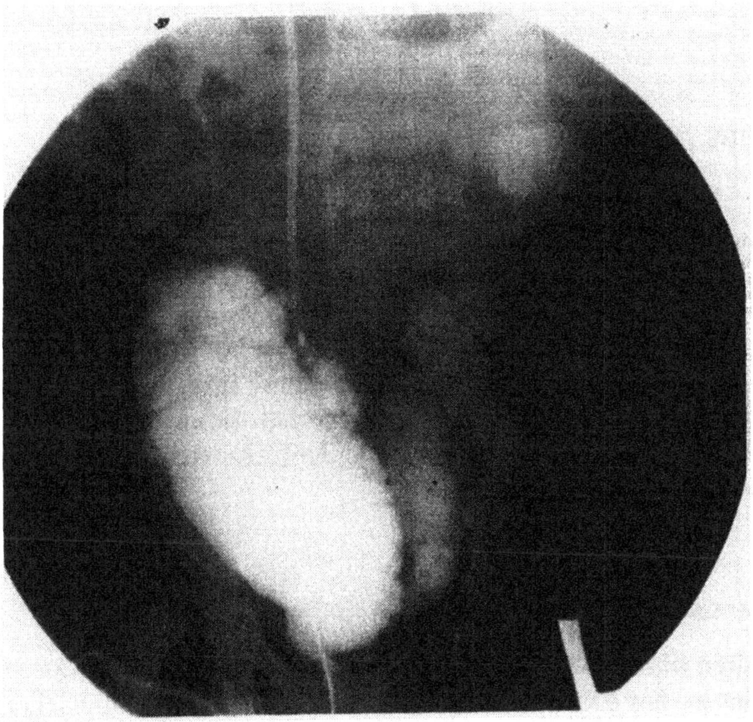

FIGURE 2.1 Micturating cysto-urethrogram in a 2-year-old child with spina bifida. Clinical details are presented in the text

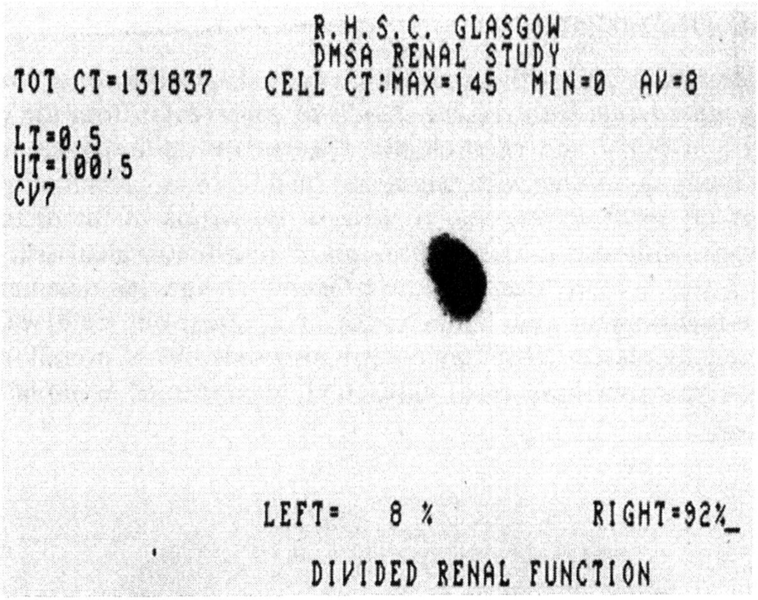

FIGURE 2.2 DMSA scan in the same 2-year-old child

Posterior urethral valves in the neonate and young infant require early diagnosis and urgent treatment.

Figure 2.3 shows an antegrade pyelogram study in a 12-year-old boy presenting with end-stage renal disease, dwarfism and a long history of recurrent urinary tract infections. Investigations in early childhood would presumably have revealed the reversible lesion of stenosis at the uretero-vesical junction. Unfortunately, he had a single kidney.

Anaemia

Children with renal failure show a normochromic normocytic anaemia similar to that observed in adults with chronic renal failure. There is a decrease in the rate of red cell production and the circulating red blood cells have a shortened life span[4]. Erythropoietin levels are low and inhibitors of erythropoietin may exist[5]. Because of poor appetite,

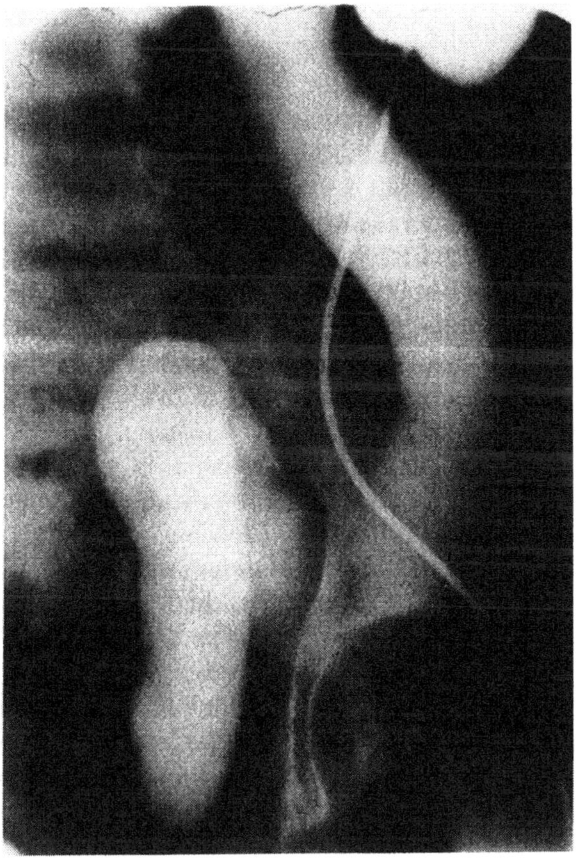

FIGURE 2.3 Antegrade pyelogram in a 12-year-old boy presenting with end-stage renal disease secondary to an obstruction at the vesicoureteric junction

intake of both iron and folic acid may be inadequate and supplements should be given. It is, however, important not to cause iron overload and the serum ferritin concentration should be measured before starting treatment. Our practice is to prescribe 1 Fefol spansule (150 mg ferrous sulphate + 0.5 mg folic acid) daily.

Renal osteodystrophy

With progressive reduction in the glomerular filtration rate, resistance to vitamin D occurs and leads to decreased absorption of calcium. Hyperphosphataemia results, causing a decrease in ionized calcium and a secondary increase in the serum parathyroid hormone concentration. These factors eventually cause the bone changes of rickets and secondary hyperparathyroidism[6]. Early recognition of renal osteodystrophy is important because deformity can occur over a short time during a period of rapid growth. It is recommended[7] that alfacalcidol ($0.05\,\mu g\,kg^{-1}\,day^{-1}$) [$1\alpha(OH)$-$D_3$] be prescribed when the glomerular filtration rate falls below $60\,ml\,min^{-1}\,1.73\,m^{-2}$. In addition, it is important that oral calcium intake is adequate, and that phosphate intake is reduced if hyperphosphataemia is present. When normophosphataemia cannot be achieved by dietary phosphate restriction alone, an oral phosphate binding agent may be necessary. Since the death of a child in 1980 with aluminium encephalopathy, calcium carbonate has been the phosphate binding agent of choice for the children on the Glasgow programme. The drug is given with feeds in the dosage necessary to reduce plasma phosphate concentration to as near the normal range as possible. Systemic acidosis must be corrected using either sodium bicarbonate capsules or Shohl's solution. The diagnosis of renal osteodystrophy is confirmed with the measurement of circulating immunoreactive parathormone (iPTH) concentrations and serial measurements are used as a guide to $1\alpha(OH)$-D_3 dosage. Radiological skeletal surveys provide only a rough guide to the diagnosis and progress. We have recently presented our experience with $1\alpha(OH)$-D_3 in renal osteodystrophy[8]. The accompanying series of X-rays (Figure 2.4) shows the effect of this conservative therapy on one child over the period of 4 years.

Nutritional disturbances

The growth and nutritional state of children with chronic renal disease can be severely disturbed. This is especially so in children with hypoplastic/dysplastic disease and with obstructive uropathy. It has been shown that better growth is achieved when children do have an

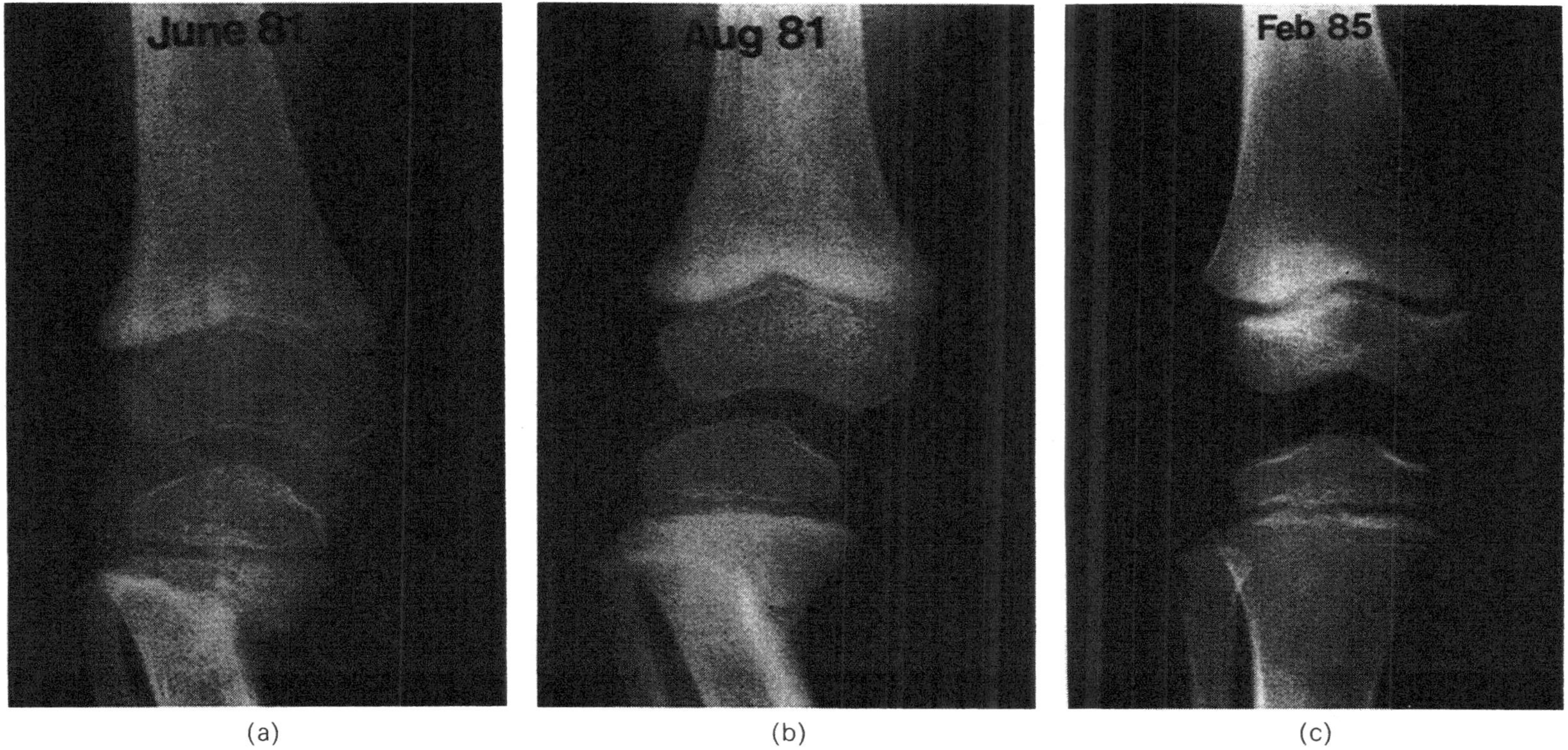

FIGURE 2.4 Anteroposterior radiographs of the right knee of a 3-year-old girl showing a fracture through the metaphysisis, (a) before treatment, (b) after 2 months, and (c) after 4 years of treatment

adequate calorie intake[9]. This demands team work between the dietitian and nephrologist as well as close supervision. Our practice is to suggest that children receive the recommended dietary allowances with calorie intakes of up to 120 Cal kg^{-1} day^{-1} in early infancy falling off to 40–50 Cal kg^{-1} day^{-1} at adolescence. Protein intake varies from 0.5 to 2.5 g kg^{-1} day^{-1} according to the GFR with calcium intakes of 500 mg to 1.5 g/day according to blood calcium levels. Fluid intake depends upon urinary output and state of hydration and varies from 200 to 2000 ml per day.

The child's nutritional status requires to be regularly assessed. Retrospective enquiry of the diet can give a rough indication of intake. Regular recordings of the height in older children and the recumbent length in younger children are advisable. Serial weights are necessary. It is important that the measurements are of good quality and taken by the same observer. The patient's height and weight are measured regularly on attendance at our clinic. We calculate the growth velocity index (GVI) as:

$$\mathrm{GVI} = \frac{\text{Actual growth velocity of patient}}{\text{Normal growth velocity for chronological age}} \times 100$$

A standard deviation score (SDS) is calculated as:

$$\mathrm{SDS} = \frac{\text{Patient's height in cm} - \text{height at 50th centile for age in cm}}{\text{Standard deviation of height for age in cm}}$$

Bone age measurements help not only in the serial assessment but in predicting the eventual height of the child. Skinfold thickness measurements are made at intervals of 3 months but they tend to vary according to the state of hydration of the child. Other units have found the plasma transferrin level as well as the total protein level useful indices of nutritional status[10].

Infants and younger children present a special problem. In recent years we have resorted to early introduction of nasogastric feeding to ensure adequate calorie intake. The effect of nasogastric feeding on six small children who had not been thriving is shown in Figure 2.5. In patients where the GFR is less than 15 ml min^{-1} 1.73 m^{-2} the blood urea may rise to levels producing symptoms of vomiting (usually above 30 mmol/l). Protein restriction of 1 g/kg is instituted. If the

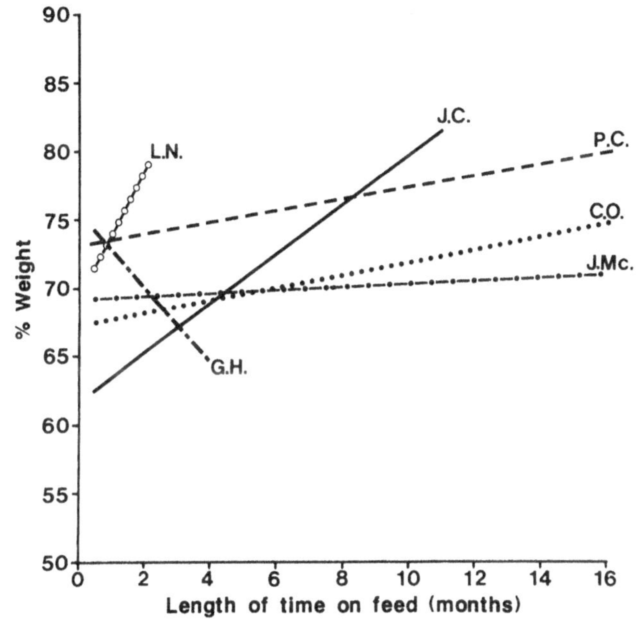

FIGURE 2.5 Effect of nasogastric feeding on the weights of six children who were failing to thrive

calorie intake can be maintained at between 120 and 150 cal/kg weight, growth can still be achieved. Relief of family tension because of 'toddler striking' as well as the elimination of the problem of poor drug compliance are advantages of nasogastric feeding. Children, however, in time become dependent on their nasogastric feed and may have to relearn their eating habits.

Correction of any systemic acidosis and normophosphataemia are important aims. By eliminating dairy products from the diet, effective phosphate reduction is usually possible; for infants, baby milks with a low phosphate content are available and reduce the need for large doses of phosphate binding agents. In general, children's diets are deficient in vitamins and it is usual practice to provide supplements. Ketovite liquid and ketovite tablets are given to all children with renal failure in our clinic.

Different units have different policies with regard to the conservative management of the young child with chronic renal failure. Some units would prefer a more active policy of early transplantation, aiming at better growth than is possible when the child is maintained on conservative treatment.

RENAL REPLACEMENT THERAPY

European experience

At least five new patients per million of the child population per year are accepted on to paediatric dialysis programmes in Europe[11]. Children most frequently present for their first treatment between 10 and 14 years of age.

The European Dialysis and Transplantation Association (EDTA) have defined the basic requirements for childrens' dialysis centres as a paediatric nephrologist, nurses experienced in the dialysis of children, a dietitian, a hospital school and a social worker. Paediatric surgery and urology are also required. There is also a need for psychiatric services and the support of a general paediatric unit. It has been shown that patient survival on dialysis, graft survival and patient survival after transplantation are better when children are treated in specialized units. Moreover, when transplantation is performed in a specialized paediatric centre the paediatrician is much more involved in the care of the patient[11].

During the last few years, the European data show that an increasing number of children, including pre-school children are being accepted for dialysis each year[11]. In general, better integration of the different types of treatment available is being achieved and this integration has contributed to better survival. A significant increase in patient survival for all treatments has been shown between 1978 and 1982. The contribution of transplantation to treatment programmes is increasing in many countries. Growth in pre-pubertal children is significantly better in transplanted than in dialysed children, especially if the serum creatinine concentration is less than 120 μmol/l; and growth after a failed transplant is better in children who were less than 6 years at the time of transplant than in older children.

In 1972 facilities first became available at the Royal Hospital for Sick Children (RHSC) Glasgow for the treatment of end-stage renal disease; 70 patients have been accepted on to the programme. Their

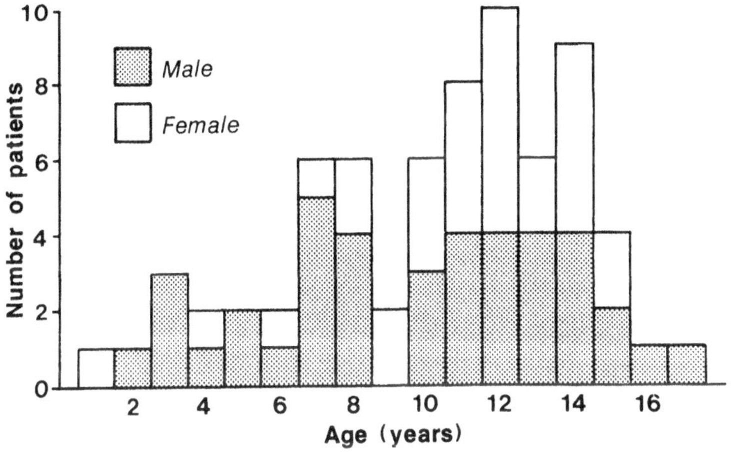

FIGURE 2.6 Age at presentation: Regular Dialysis Programme, RHSC, Glasgow

ages range from 2 months to 16 years (Figure 2.6). The underlying diseases responsible for the renal failure in these children are shown in Table 2.1. Malformations of the kidney and urinary tract, including reflux nephropathy and congenital hypoplastic/dysplastic disease, accounted for most. Of the glomerular diseases, Henoch–Schonlein nephritis predominated. Nephronopthisis was the commonest of the genetically transmitted diseases and other vascular diseases were uncommon.

Indications for dialysis

The indications for starting dialysis treatment vary. Some children require urgent and regular therapy because of hyperkalaemia which is uncontrolled either by dietary restriction or ion exchange resin. Others present with acute pulmonary oedema and need fluid removal. A child who has stable renal insufficiency may develop acute or chronic renal failure following an infective illness. In general, the history is of progressive tiredness, listlessness, itch and loss of appetite and there is time available to consider the possible different options. When the

TABLE 2.1 Causes of primary renal disease leading to end-stage renal failure, Royal Hospital for Sick Children, Glasgow, 1972–1987 (70 patients)

	No.	*% of total*
Malformations of the kidney and urinary tract	35	50
Reflux nephropathy/pyelonephritis	12	17.16
Malformative uropathies	10	14.3
Hypoplasia, dysplasia	13	18.59
Glomerular diseases	20	28.6
Henoch-Schonlein	8	11.44
Focal, segmental glomerulosclerosis	5	7.15
Membranoproliferative	2	2.86
Others, unclassified	5	7.15
Genetically transmitted disease	11	15.73
Nephronopthisis	6	8.58
Cystinosis	4	5.72
Oxalosis	1	1.43
Vascular diseases	2	2.86
Haemolytic uraemic syndrome	1	1.43
Cortical necrosis	1	1.43
Miscellaneous	2	2.86
Bilateral tumour	1	1.43
Interstitial nephritis	1	1.43

child is about to start a dialysis programme, attendance at a special clinic enables the patient and family to hear the experience of other patients on the different types of treatment available. Often the child or adolescent has no difficulty in choosing either regular haemodialysis therapy (RDT) or continuous ambulatory peritoneal dialysis (CAPD) and unless there are contra-indications, the form of treatment selected by the child and his family is accepted by the unit. The staff of the unit then partner the patient in his management. Because the waiting time for renal transplantation is prolonged (30 months on average), haemodialysis is the preferred treatment in RHSC, Glasgow. If arrangements are in hand for a live donor transplant then CAPD is preferable since it is a satisfactory treatment in the short term. Our experience would correspond to that of the European data[11] confirming that CAPD has many limitations as a long-term therapy.

Vascular access

The Cimino Brescia radiocephalic fistula remains the best method of vascular access. It is achievable, however, only in children over 15 kg even when the expertise of a paediatric vascular surgeon is available. In children under this weight, a brachial cephalic anastomosis can be created in the cubital fossa for long-term use. We have also used arteriovenous groin loops successfully; the femoral artery is linked to the femoral vein with the synthetic material, polytetrafluoroethylene (PTFE). Often the paediatric vascular surgeon has to be creative and devise different methods of vascular access in the compromised child.

Arteriovenous fistulas require time to mature before they are suitable for haemodialysis needles and a child may need temporary vascular access. The introduction of subclavian vein cannulation has been a significant development in recent years[12]. Using the Seldinger technique, a polyurethane catheter is introduced percutaneously into the superior vena cava via the subclavicular approach to the subclavian vein. Haemodialysis can be instituted within 1–2 h following presentation to the hospital. For more permanent vascular access the catheter can be buried subcutaneously (Figure 2.7). The common complication is infection, localized at the exit site and sometimes accompanied by bacteraemia or septicaemia. As traumatic pneumothorax is possible, a chest X-ray should be performed after insertion. Subclavian catheters produce acceptable blood flow for dialysis. Although flow may alter with position, the technique does offer a relatively safe and efficient method of obtaining either temporary or sustained haemodialysis in children.

Regular haemodialysis therapy

The basic principles and procedures of haemodialysis in children are the same as for adults. Life for the child on RDT is complex (Table 2.2) and it is important that their treatment requirements should be

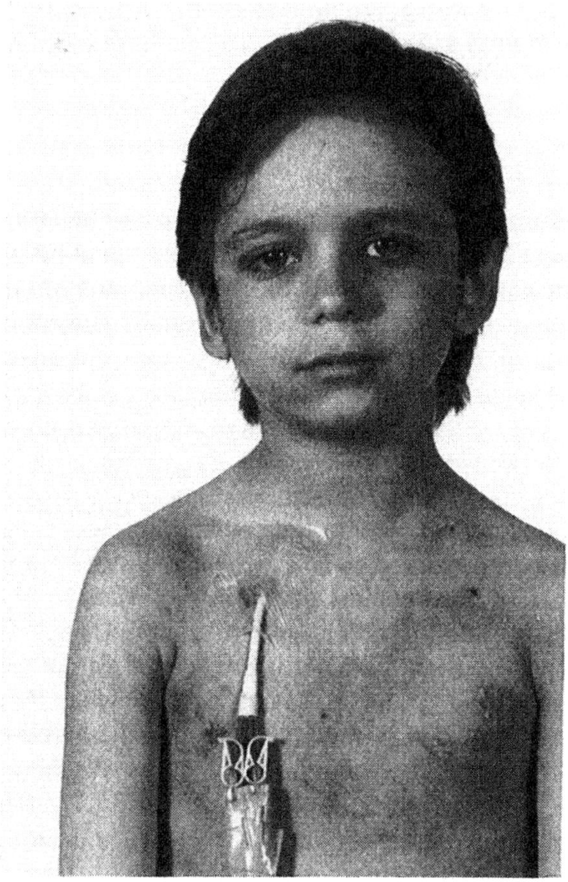

FIGURE 2.7 Double lumen subclavian cannula

modified to meet their individual requirements.

Paediatric dialysers with priming volumes varying from 20 to 150 ml and membrane surface areas from 0.23 to 1 m^2 are available. Special paediatric lines have volumes varying between 35 and 75 ml. The dialyser, the lines and the blood flow rate require to be individually prescribed for each patient. The volume of the extracorporeal blood circuit should be less than 10% of the patient's blood volume (blood volume = 80 ml/kg body weight). In patients weighing less than 10 kg a blood flow rate of less than 75 ml/min is advisable; from 10 to 20 kg

TABLE 2.2 Life for a child on RDT

(1)	Diet
(2)	Fluid restriction
(3)	Fistula cannulation
(4)	Three times weekly dialysis
(5)	Adjustment to low Hb level
(6)	Growth failure
(7)	Delayed puberty
(8)	Patient/family stress

less than 150 ml/min; in those over 20 kg up to 250 ml/min. The ratio of the dialyser surface area to patient surface area should be around 0.75 and this provides a useful guide to the size of the dialyser which should be used. Heparin must be given during haemodialysis to prevent the blood clotting in the dialyser and extracorporeal circulation (Table 2.3).

Regional heparinization is indicated after surgery, if coagulation is abnormal, and when there is thrombocytopenia or bleeding within the previous 48 h. If the patient is being dialysed pre-operatively, regional heparinization is also advisable. The smaller the child on dialysis, the greater are the chances of dialysis disequilibrium or

TABLE 2.3 Heparinization schedule

Systemic

(a) *Initial heparin dosage*

Weight	*Dose*
5–15 kg	50–250 units
15–25 kg	250–500 units
25–35 kg	500–750 units
35–55 kg	750–1000 units

(b) *Maintenance dose*
100 units/kg for 5 h haemodialysis. 60% of total dose given by infusion over the first 2.5 h.

Regional
800–1000 units heparin/hour + 8–10 mg protamine/h

hypovolaemia. The symptoms are nausea, vomiting, headache and dizziness; convulsions may sometimes occur during or after dialysis. To reduce the risks of these unwanted complications, salt and water should be removed by ultrafiltration gradually and evenly during the course of dialysis. Ultrafiltration modules are, therefore, a development of significant benefit to the paediatrician. In addition, the introduction of bicarbonate dialysis has, in our experience, significantly reduced symptoms during dialysis. Most children receive between 12 and 15 h dialysis per week, but the range varies from 6 to 20 h.

Infants and smaller children on haemodialysis present a special problem. Adequate sedation is indicated and arm restrainers are required in infants. Frequent recordings of vital signs are necessary. Straight connection on to dialysis lines without depleting the child's intravascular volume prevents initial hypotension. Changes in flow rate and ultrafiltration rate are made with caution and the use of an ultrafiltration module with continuous read-out of fluid removal is indicated. Once the difficulties of the technical procedure are overcome even very young infants under 6 months old remain well and happy on RDT.

Home haemodialysis

Before the introduction of CAPD as a home-based treatment for the child with chronic renal failure, home haemodialysis was considered the optimum therapy when the waiting time for renal transplant was prolonged. Even at present, it offers the best chance of rehabilitation for the child facing haemodialysis in the long term, e.g. failed transplant with high level of cytotoxic antibodies. School attendance, family life, social interaction are all improved on home haemodialysis compared to a hospital-based programme. In addition, it remains the treatment of choice for families living in outlying areas where CAPD is not possible. Usually training of the child and one parent is undertaken. Experience of setting up and dismantling the machine gives the confidence to proceed to managing the dialysis treatment itself. The difficult step is that of fistula cannulation: usually the child opts to self-cannulate but often the parent takes on that responsibility. We have been surprised to find success in unlikely family situations, e.g.

single parent, socially deprived, two siblings affected, etc. Once trained, the patient opts to continue dialysis in the home whenever necessary, e.g. after a failed transplant. Home haemodialysis may involve the family in a change of home, upset to other siblings and heavy financial implications. An important pre-requisite for a home dialysis programme is the support – nursing, technical and practical – from the dialysis unit.

Continuous ambulatory peritoneal dialysis

Since the description of the method by Popovich *et al.* in 1976[13], CAPD has been an increasingly popular method of routine dialysis for children with end-stage renal disease. It is a home-based, pain-free, ambulant treatment and offers improved quality of life for the patient and the family. There is effective control of the biochemical abnormalities associated with uraemia and some improvement in anaemia, but the life style for the child remains complex (Table 2.4). Between

TABLE 2.4 Life for a child on CAPD

(1)	Diet
(2)	Permanent abdominal cannula
(3)	Cycle changes, 6 hourly, 7 days
(4)	Complications: peritonitis, cannula
(5)	Dwarfism, delayed puberty
(6)	Adjustment to low Hb level
(7)	Patient/family strain

1979 and 1985, 26 children were commenced on CAPD in RHSC, Glasgow. There were 13 males and 13 females with an age range of 0.25 to 16.7 years. The mean age at initiation of CAPD was 9.8 years. The length of time on CAPD was between 1 and 40 months, with a mean time of 12.9 months per patient. The mean body weight at initiation of CAPD was 22.8 kg with a range of 5.1–44 kg. The reasons for commencing CAPD are shown in Table 2.5.

TABLE 2.5 CAPD

Reason for CAPD	*Number of patients*
Patient size	13
Patient and family preference	9
Vascular access difficulties	6
Non-compliance on haemodialysis	3
Distance from hospital	1
Idiopathic ascites	1
Intellectual retardation	1

Technique

All patients were dialysed through a permanent indwelling catheter, which was tailored to the size of the child and inserted surgically through a small laparotomy. Initially double cuff Tenckhoff catheters were used but because of infections in the catheter tunnel one cuff paediatric Tenckhoff catheters were selected. Since 1984 Goretex cannulas have replaced the Tenckhoff catheter for routine use (Figure 2.8). Since that time our postoperative procedure has been to flush the cannula on return from theatre until the effluent is free of blood and then flush with small volumes of dialysate daily for the next 2 weeks. This practice has reduced the incidence of leakage around the catheter insertion site and tunnel infections. Patients with symptoms of uraemia require haemodialysis to tide them over this period. Training can commence, however, and both the parent and child are instructed in the technique. The child's home can be assessed and alterations carried out in preparation for his discharge from hospital. CAPD is performed using 0.5, 0.75 or 1 litre bags of commercially available dialysate (Travenol). All patients have four or five exchange cycles daily using dialysate containing either 13.6 g glucose/l, 22.7 g/l or 38.6 g/l dialysate fluid. In 14 children the exchanges are performed by the parents and in 10 patients aged over 12 years exchanges are undertaken by the patients themselves. There are no dietary or fluid restrictions but a high protein intake is encouraged.

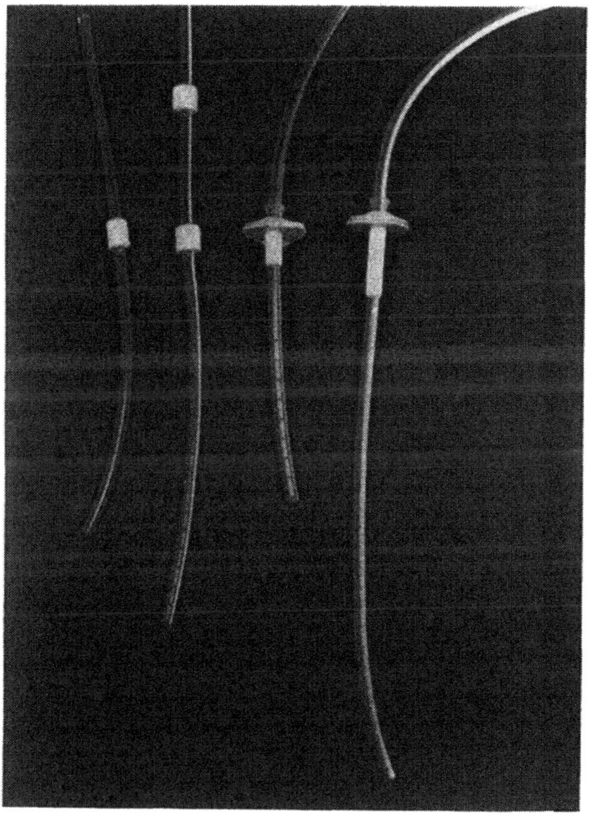

FIGURE 2.8 Single cuff Tenckhoff, double cuff Tenckhoff and Goretex PD cannulas

Biochemistry

The accompanying graphs (Figure 2.9) illustrate the biochemical features of the children on CAPD and indicate the time required for this treatment to become effective. Plasma urea was controlled between 20 and 25 mmol/l and creatinine between 600 and 700 μmol/l. The mean total protein concentrations were within normal limits. The mean albumin concentrations were below the normal range but tended to rise during time on CAPD. Plasma calcium concentrations were low at the start of treatment but rose to within the normal range although

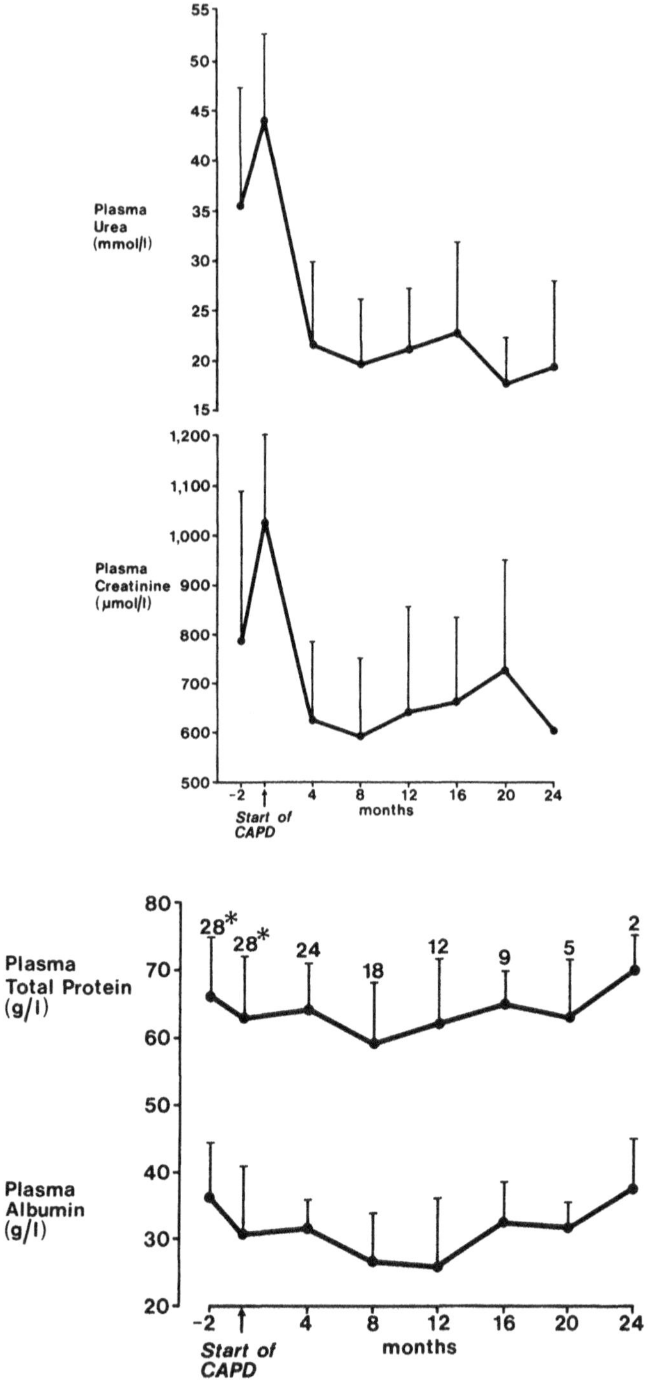

FIGURE 2.9 Serial biochemistry in 26 CAPD patients

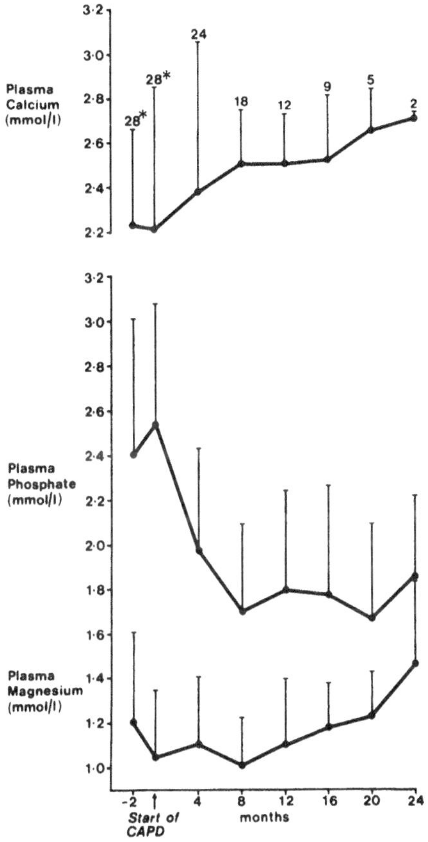
Plasma Calcium (mmol/l)
3·2
3·0
2·8
2·6
2·4
2·2
28*
28*
24
18
12
9
5
2
Plasma Phosphate (mmol/l)
3·2
3·0
2·8
2·6
2·4
2·2
2·0
1·8
1·6
1·4
1·2
1·0
Plasma Magnesium (mmol/l)
-2
4
8
12
16
20
24
Start of CAPD
months

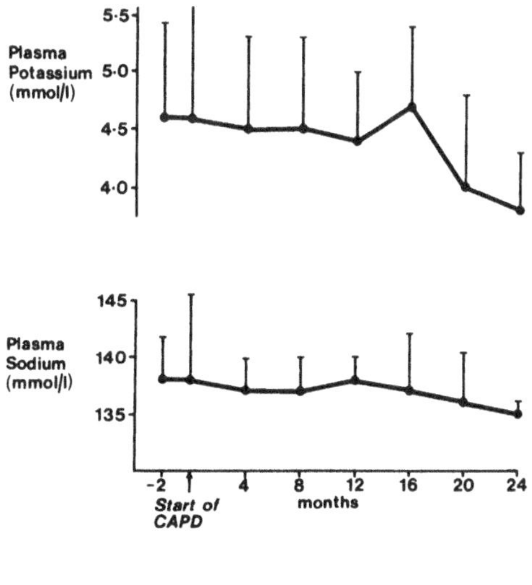
Plasma Potassium (mmol/l)
5·5
5·0
4·5
4·0
Plasma Sodium (mmol/l)
145
140
135
-2
4
8
12
16
20
24
Start of CAPD
months

phosphate levels remained persistently high. Plasma potassium concentrations fell gradually over 2 years to within the normal range.

Haematology

Haemoglobin levels showed an increase in all patients with a mean of 6.29 g/dl at the start and 8.43 g/dl at the end of treatment (Figure 2.10). The mean blood transfusion requirement was 0.3 units per patient month.

Growth and nutrition

The patients were classified into three groups according to their growth velocity index (GVI). The GVI was defined as 'normal' when it was 80%, 'fair' between 50 and 80% and 'poor' at 50% of normal. Eleven

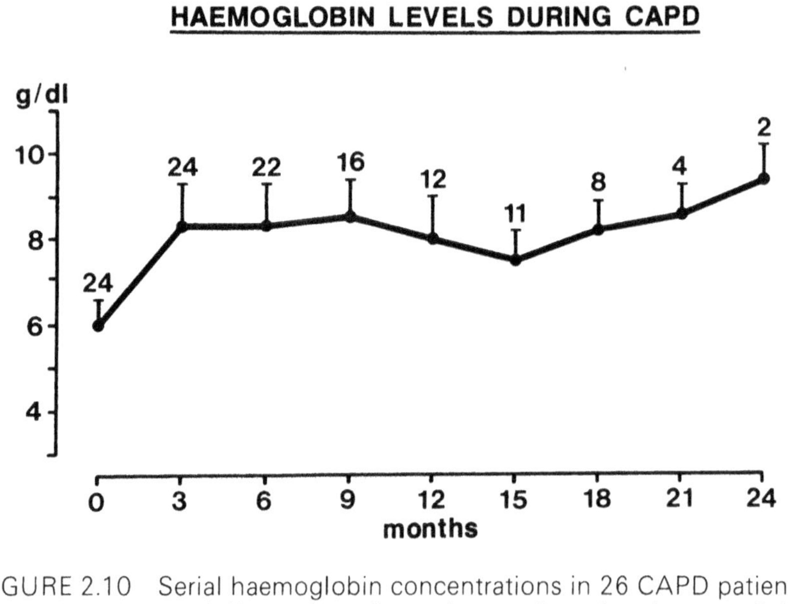

FIGURE 2.10 Serial haemoglobin concentrations in 26 CAPD patients. The numbers at each line point refer to the number of patients available for study

out of 24 patients with serial measurements available had normal growth (45%), eight had poor growth (35%) and five had fair growth (21%) as determined by their GVI. Plasma urea, creatinine, bicarbonate and haemoglobin values did not differ significantly between the patients who had normal growth and those with impaired growth.

Education

Seventeen of the 26 patients were able to return to their normal schools and they seemed to cope well. Two mentally handicapped children went to special schools and a further four patients attended special school due to physical handicap. Three patients were under school age.

Complications

The complications are shown in Table 2.6. Peritonitis was the main problem (Figure 2.11). Our criteria for the diagnosis of peritonitis

TABLE 2.6 Complications of CAPD

Infection	
Recurrent/persistent peritonitis	11
Abscess formation	3
Recurrent exit site infection	9
Technical	
Leakage	10
Blockage	4
Mobility or disconnection	6
Others	
Poor control of hypertension	9
Hypotension	3
Fluid overload	3
Convulsions	10
Abdominal hernia	5
Psychological problems	1

were cloudy peritoneal fluid with abdominal pain and positive cytur test. There was an incidence of one episode of peritonitis every 3.5 patient months. Coagulase negative staphylococci, and *Staphylococcus aureus* were the most common isolates, together accounting for 46.4% of all episodes (Table 2.7). Culture negative peritonitis was relatively frequent accounting for 27.8% of the episodes. Fungal peritonitis occurred on six occasions and candida species was responsible for the infection in four cases. One patient died during CAPD from *S. aureus* peritonitis and septicaemia. Postmortem examination

TABLE 2.7 Culture results from 97 episodes of peritonitis in 26 patients on CAPD

Micro-organisms	*No. of episodes*	%
Gram +ve		
Coagulase-neg. staph.	25	25.8
Staph. aureus	20	20.6
Strep. viridans	3	3.1
Gp. A. strep.	1	1.0
Gram −ve		
Ps. aeruginosa	1	1.0
Pr. mirabilis	1	1.0
Ent. cloacae	1	1.0
Citro. freundii	1	1.0
H. influenzae	1	1.0
Mixed		
2 Gram −ve	4	4.1
2 Gram +ve	4	4.1
1 Gram +ve and 1 Gram −ve	2	2.1
Fungi		
Candida albicans	3	3.1
Candida glabrata	1	1.0
Cryptococcus laurentii	1	1.0
Saccharomyces cerevisiae	1	1.0
Nil		
No growth	27	27.8
Total	97	100

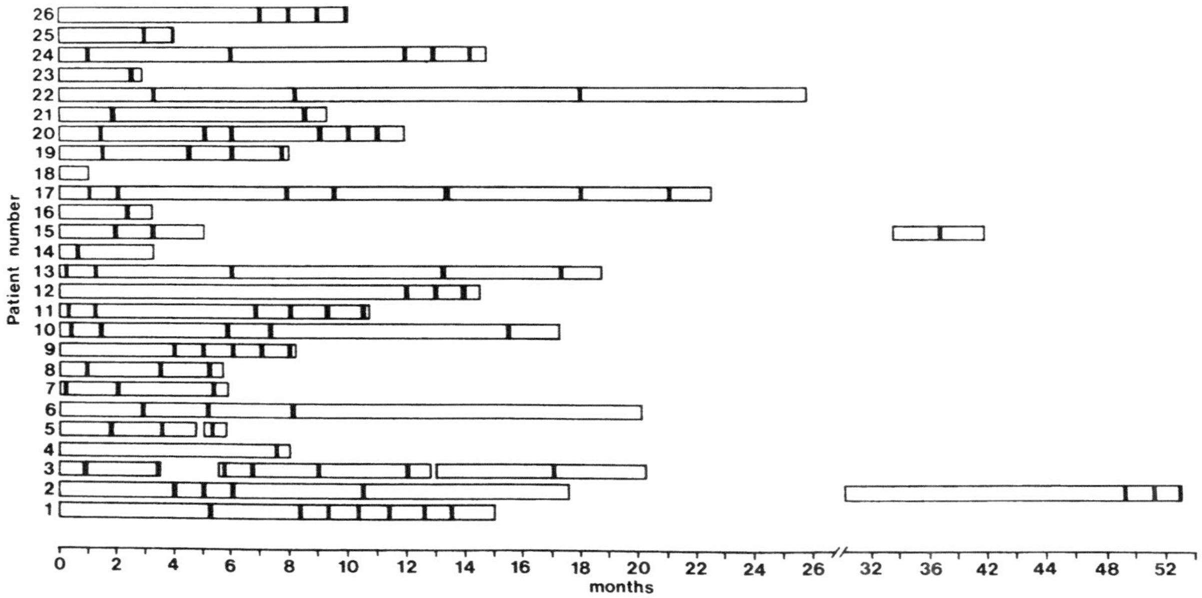

FIGURE 2.11 Number of episodes of peritonitis in 26 patients on CAPD

revealed an encapsulated staphylococcal muscle abscess in addition to peritonitis.

Our initial choice of best guess therapy early in the series was cephamandol with the addition of gentamicin or tobramicin for Gram negative organisms. In the light of experience with poor clinical results and increased resistance to cephamandol, vancomicin is now the first choice antibiotic with netilmicin being added to cover the Gram negative bacteria. Therapy is given as follows:

> Netilmicin 2.5 mg/kg loading dose intramuscularly, then netilmicin 5 mg/l dialysate fluid. Vancomicin 250 mg/l for the first exchange, then 25 mg/l dialysate fluid. Both drugs are given for 7–10 days.

In fungal peritonitis the most important factor in treatment was early catheter removal, after a short primary course of intraperitoneal antifungal drugs.

In addition to peritonitis, technical problems relating to the cannula were observed. Figure 2.12 shows a micturating cystogram in a child on CAPD complaining of suprapubic discomfort. The contrast is present in the peritoneal catheter which has entered the bladder following pressure necrosis.

Fourteen patients required antihypertensive therapy. Convulsions occurred in ten patients and six of these had a previous history of convulsions. Two out of the ten were hypertensive prior to the fit. Convulsions in the others were probably due to the disequilibrium syndrome. Figure 2.13 shows the progress and outcome of the 26 CAPD patients. Eight received cadaveric transplants 3–40 months after starting treatment and two received live donor transplants. Ten patients were transferred to haemodialysis, four died and five remained on CAPD. The study demonstrates that there was a significant mortality in this group of patients, that CAPD does have limitations as a therapy for long-term use, and that alternative therapies are required.

RENAL TRANSPLANTATION

It is now clear that renal transplantation offers the best chance of rehabilitation for the child with end-stage renal disease. If the graft functions well, growth, puberty, general well-being and freedom from

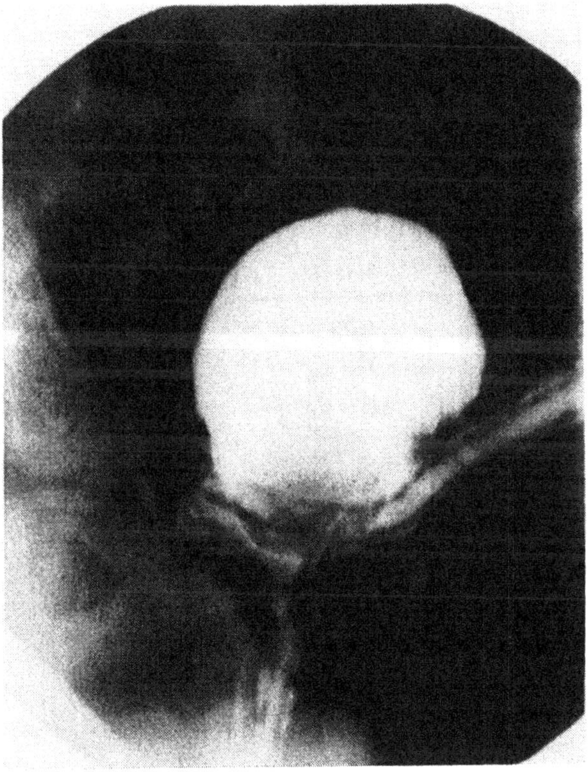

FIGURE 2.12 Micturating cystogram in a 5-year-old child on CAPD: see text for details

intensive hospital supervision all follow. Improvement in graft survival during the last 5 years has been well demonstrated from data available to the EDTA[11] (Table 2.8). When the child starts regular dialysis therapy, preparations begin for his inclusion in the pool of patients awaiting a cadaveric graft.

Immunology

If the offer of a live donor transplant is available, arrangements are made for the assessment of the donor in the adult transplant unit. The value of HLA-A and -B matching in live donor transplantation is

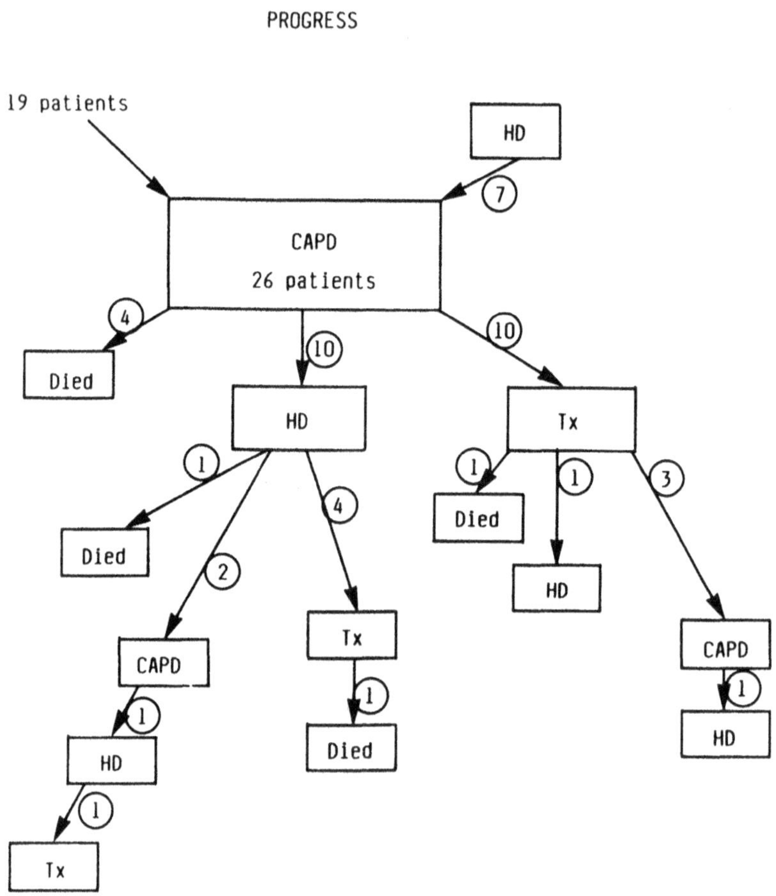

FIGURE 2.13 Origin and progress of 26 patients on CAPD

clear. In cadaver renal transplantation there are reports demonstrating a correlation between HLA-A and -B matching and improved cadaver renal allograft outcome[14] but many large studies have failed to confirm this association. Matching for HLA-DR antigen in cadaver renal transplantation does, however, appear to correlate well with allograft outcome[15]. ABO and Rh blood groups and HLA-A, -B and -DR antigens are known in all potential transplant recipients. Their sera is checked regularly for lymphocytotoxic antibodies. Pretransplant

TABLE 2.8 Improvement in graft survival during the last 5 years (EDTA data)

	Sample size	*% graft survival*		
		6 month	*1 year*	*5 years*
Before 1.1.78				
CT	430	67	61	45
LRT	188	81	79	(55)
After 1.1.78				
CT	586	75	69	50
LRT	210	89	85	(67)

CT = cadaver transplant; LRT = live related transplant

blood transfusion has been shown to improve graft survival[16] and it is our practice to give 3 aliquots of blood to each potential recipient.

Immunosuppressive therapy

Since 1983, cyclosporin has replaced azathioprine as the immunosuppressive agent of choice in renal transplantation. As in Europe[11], our experience suggests that fewer rejection episodes occur when cyclosporin is given. The rejection episodes, however, are more difficult to detect clinically; frequently the only sign is a rise in serum creatinine. The optimal dose of the drug is still not clear. Smaller children require a relatively higher dosage to maintain therapeutic levels than older children. We continue to prescribe steroid along with cyclosporin. Nephrotoxicity has been common in our experience and it is important to have access to frequent cyclosporin assays. With reduction in dose, the nephrotoxicity is usually reversible. Side-effects experienced by the children, tremor, hirsutism and gum hypertrophy, can persist after the drug is withdrawn. Our immunosuppressive regime is shown in Table 2.9.

TABLE 2.9 Transplant immunosuppression

Cyclosporin

Pre-operatively: 15 mg/kg
Day 1 to day 7: 15 mg kg^{-1} day^{-1}
Day 8 to day 21: 10 mg kg^{-1} day^{-1}
Reduction after this stage, dependent on graft function and blood levels.
Therapeutic range 150–400 μg/ml (radioimmunoassay)

Prednisolone

(a) *Cadaver*

	1 week	3 weeks	6 weeks	9 weeks post-transplant
	3	1	0.5	0.25 mg kg^{-1} day^{-1}

(b) *Living related*

3 days pretransplant: 3 mg kg^{-1} day^{-1}

	1 week	3 weeks	6 weeks	9 weeks post-transplant
1/2 HLA	3	1	0.5	0.25 mg kg^{-1} day^{-1}
HLA identical	3	0.5	0.25	0.18–0.25

Acute rejection episodes

Occurring within the first month:

Methyl prednisolone 600 mg m^{-2} day^{-1} is infused intravenously for 3 consecutive days, followed by a further three doses on alternate days should this be required. If the rejection episode occurs after the first month after transplant, oral anti-rejection therapy is given as 3 mg/kg prednisolone per day until the rejection episode is controlled.

Perioperative management

Ideally the transplant surgeon, paediatric nephrologist and anaesthetist work together. It is important to document the patient's weight and pretransplant urine volume. If he has been treated on CAPD the latest peritoneal culture report should be available. If haemodialysis is required, biochemical correction should be aimed at without any significant weight loss in order to prevent volume depletion and poor graft perfusion. Blood is made available and the patient receives his pre-operative dose of cyclosporin.

During surgery, on intermittent positive pressure ventilation

(IPPV), the intravascular volume is maintained steady with a central venous pressure (CVP) between 10 and 15 cm of water. Intraoperative volume losses are replaced with a combination of packed cells and plasma, maintaining adequate blood pressure. 15 min prior to the vascular anastomosis, methyl prednisolone 600 mg/m^2 is given intravenously and an intravenous dopamine infusion ($5\,\mu g\,kg^{-1}\,min^{-1}$) started. If there is no diuresis within 30–60 min, intravenous frusemide is given over 10–15 min in the dose of 2–5 mg/kg. With the child off IPPV, CVP should be maintained between 5 and 10 cm of water.

Postoperatively, hourly urine volumes are replaced as 0.45% sodium chloride. Electrolyte measurements are carried out 4-hourly. Insensible loss is replaced as 0.225% saline and 5% dextrose and abnormal fluid losses by 0.9% sodium chloride. Fluid balance is calculated on a 12-hour basis and the patient is weighed daily. Cyclosporin and prednisolone are prescribed daily according to the regime shown (Table 2.5). Technetium DTPA perfusion scan is carried out 24–48 h after transplantation.

Assessment of progress

Progress is assessed by means of accurate urine volume recordings, 8–12 hourly biochemical checks, and DTPA technetium 99m perfusion scan every 2–3 days. It is our practice to work out the perfusion index[4] as it is helpful to have serial perfusion index readings available to diagnose rejection as early as possible. Ultrasound examination as a base line is a routine within the first few days after operation.

Complications

Acute tubular necrosis

When the patient is anuric and the initial perfusion study demonstrates blood flow to the kidney, acute tubular necrosis (ATN) is a possible diagnosis. It is particularly likely in allografts with a prolonged period of warm ischaemia. Anuria may be present from the time of surgery or urinary output may decrease gradually during the subsequent 24 h. It is important to be aware of this 'honeymoon diuresis' situation, because of the need for caution in administering fluids and the possibility of sudden acute pulmonary oedema. In acute tubular necrosis, an isotope perfusion scan will generally show adequate perfusion but little or no excretion of isotope.

Rejection

The most common complication of renal transplantation is graft rejection. In hyperacute rejection the clinical signs are clear. There is sudden onset of fever, graft pain, malaise, hypertension and anuria. When rejection is less acute the clinical signs may be of listlessness, irritability and graft tenderness, the signs being associated with a rise in serum creatinine with or without increased protein excretion in the urine. Rejection often occurs at a time when the child has infection in the urinary tract or elsewhere. The diagnosis can be difficult and may only be made following the response of the patient to antirejection therapy. Serial isotope renograms may be helpful. During rejection (or cyclosporin toxicity) isotope excretion decreases and the perfusion index[17] deteriorates. The rise in the perfusion index corresponds to the fall in renal blood flow which occurs during rejection. Graft biopsy is indicated in some situations, to distinguish between ATN, rejection and cyclosporin nephrotoxicity.

Urological complications

Surgical problems after transplantation are more common in children than in adults because of their small size or because of the small size of the donor kidney. Urinary leaks can occur following surgical reconstruction of the urinary system. Clinically the child presents with abdominal distension and oliguria while the isotope scan may show leakage of isotope into the abdominal cavity. Stenosis at the ureterovesical junction can also occur in a child who may show an elevation in serum creatinine concentration and some decrease in urinary output but no other signs of clinical rejection. Ultrasound examination generally confirms the diagnosis. Surgical correction is required.

Renal artery stenosis

In recent years more donor kidneys have been available from the preschool age group and a significant incidence of renal artery stenosis has been reported in recipients when donors were less than 2 years of age[18]. In any child with sudden onset of hypertension or hypertensive encephalopathy, post-transplant arteriography is indicated to confirm or exclude a diagnosis of renal artery stenosis.

Recurrence of primary disease

The presence of proteinuria occurring in transplanted patients whose primary disease was focal segmental glomerulosclerosis raises the possibility of recurrence of their primary disease. Reports[19] suggest that the shorter the duration of the original disease, the higher the risk of developing recurrence. Older children are more at risk of recurrence than younger.

Psychosocial factors

General

The task of the renal unit team is to ensure not only satisfactory physical growth from infancy to adult life for the patient but also to ensure normal psychological maturity (Figure 2.14). The child is part of a family unit in which relationships will be influenced by the patient's illness. If the family can be supported through the various stages of acceptance of the implications of the illness there will be normal psychosocial development.

When the child and family first hear the news of a serious illness their reaction is as with any other stressful event. There may be signs of denial. The tendency is to blame themselves or others for the child's illness. They may collude with the non-compliance of their child to therapy or to diet and ignore advice given. They may seek support from different members of staff, causing confusion and difficulties in communication among the staff. Many parents remain in this stage for some years. They can become knowledgeable and acquainted with

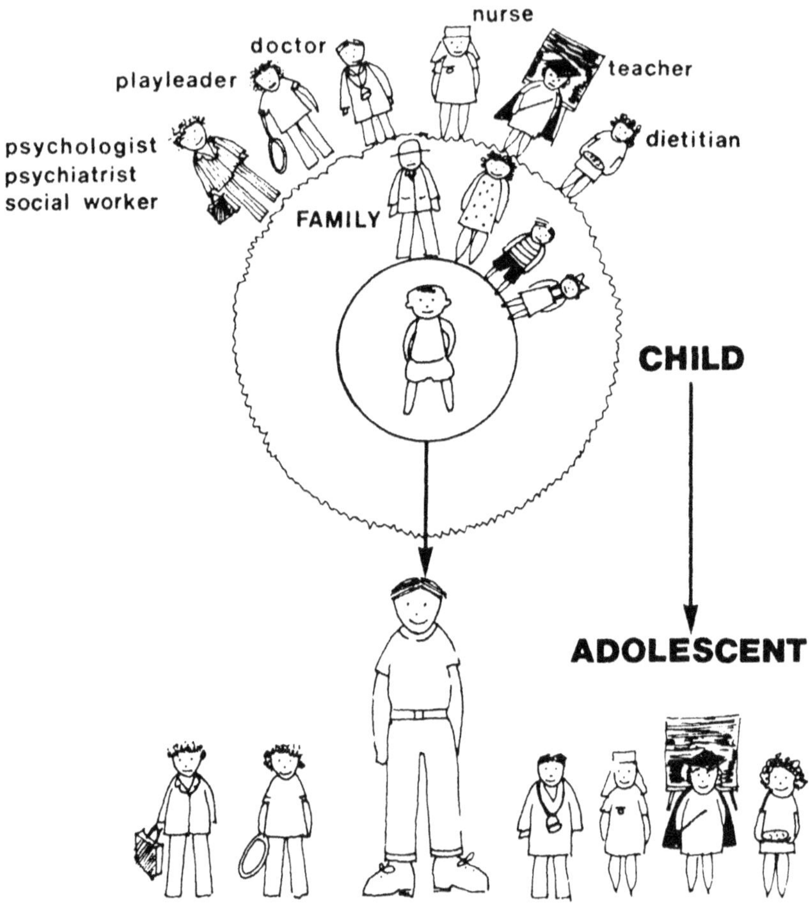

FIGURE 2.14 Managing the child with chronic illness

the illness and the different techniques available and can set themselves up as experts, offering information and guidance to new parents. Often the phase of denial gives way to reactions of anger as parents realize the seriousness of their child's illness. They may then find difficulty in trusting staff, become possessive of their child and actively interfere with the child's treatment. Firm clear guidelines to staff, parents and child are required. Parents may continue to overprotect their child in this way even through adolescence, preventing the normal independence which develops at this time of life.

In general, however, with adequate information, support and opportunity to exchange experiences with other parents, families do move to a stage of accepting the seriousness of the child's illness. Often parents who have initially offered themselves as possible transplant donors withdraw their offer but become more trusting and co-operate with the child's treatment programme. At this stage important decisions regarding type of therapy, timing of transplant, etc. can be made by the parents in conjunction with the paediatric staff.

Attitudes to illness

In order to understand more fully the needs of patients and families, we have carried out two studies[20,21] on the attitudes of staff, parents and patients to illness. We have also used the data we obtained to review our treatment policies. In the first study 13 staff members made up of different disciplines, 13 mothers and 13 children were asked to rate their feelings with regard to the illness of the children. Ten scales were provided as shown (Table 2.10) and their opinions were recorded by marking a X on a line drawn between two opposing attitudes. The results of the study allowed us to assess the coping ability of the different groups. When we looked at how staff members, mothers and

TABLE 2.10 Questionnaire: Attitudes to childhood renal failure

Negative attitude	10 9 8 7 6 5 4 3 2 1 0	*Positive attitude*
Sick	______	Healthy
Sad	______	Happy
Not going	______	Going to school
Few pals	______	Many pals
Tired	______	Full of energy
Look sick	______	Look well
Not normal	______	Lead normal life

patients were coping with illness, we found that children and staff coped well but mothers less well. We saw the need to offer more support to mothers as part of our treatment programme. When the future was considered, however, mothers and children were more optimistic than staff. Staff were in general less hopeful because of their experience of morbidity and mortality. This result demonstrated the staff's need for continual encouragement.

Turning to the different treatment options available, all groups, i.e. staff, mothers and patients, chose transplantation as the preferable mode of treatment when present and future well-being was considered. A home-based treatment programme, e.g. home haemodialysis or CAPD, was judged better than a hospital-based treatment programme.

In the second study, an attempt was again made to assess attitudes – but particularly denial as a defence mechanism in patients and their parents. In addition assessments of parental depression and the effect this might have on the child's treatment were made. Our results confirmed that in the children and also in some of the parents denial was being used as a defence mechanism. It was considered, however, that the effect was not detrimental but supportive, helping the parents and patients to cope. Depression was noted, but did not seem to have any significant effect on the child's illness.

Adolescence

The adolescent with chronic renal failure presents a special problem in management. In this age group the individual often does not want to be dependent and yet shies away from isolation. Physical changes in the body can be a problem but the delayed growth and lack of puberty experienced by patients makes them feel different from their peers. The staff are important to teenagers, helping them with the transition. It is a challenge to staff to change from their more usual parent/child approach to managing the adolescent. It is important that they are firm and absorb the tensions without feeling hurt. Many of our patients in the past have found the transition from the paediatric dialysis programme to an adult dialysis programme difficult. We, therefore, create a programme of transfer for each patient, between the ages of 13 and 16 years. The patient has an initial visit to the adult nephrology unit with a view to meeting the staff and making relationships with adult patients. The patient then, after a variable length of time, chooses to change his place of therapy. Ideally this takes place at a time when his physical condition is stable. Patients who experience renal failure for the first time during adolescence have a more difficult time than others. The most helpful approach is to involve the adolescent and his family as fully as possible in his treatment programme.

Renal Unit team

The child with chronic renal disease requires help to continue developing life apart from his treatment and his time in hospital. School is especially important, as well as the broader aspects of education, e.g. physical exercise, social life, developing of talents, attention to holidays, interaction with peers. An active programme should be planned and offered to the children. It is important, therefore, to develop the team aspects of the multidisciplinary management necessary for children with renal failure and their families. Doctors, nurses, dietitian, teacher, social worker, technical and administrative staff are all in close contact with families. All have unique and important roles. Problems of territory naturally arise. The different authority bases from which all the disciplines come can lead to difficulties in team identity and co-ordination. A regular meeting for staff communication is essential. Recurring difficulties with communication are natural and interdisciplinary rivalry with a continuing search for clarification of roles occurs. There is a need for clear guidelines on treatment policies and decision making. We have found the presence of a child and family psychiatrist and child psychologist to be helpful. In time, primary care staff acquire skills and expertise from these specialists. The health of the Renal Unit team can be determined by its ability to evaluate its practice.

References

1. Potter, D., Larsen, D. and Leumann, E. (1970). Treatment of chronic uraemia in childhood. *Paediatrics*, **46**, 678
2. Fine, R. N., Depalma, J. R. and Lieberman, E. (1968). Extended haemodialysis in children with chronic renal failure. *J. Paediatr.*, **73**, 706
3. Chan, J. C. M., Gopelrud, J. M., Papadopoulou, Z. L. and Movello, A. C. (1981). Kidney failure in childhood. *Int. J. Paediatr. Nephrol.*, **2**, 201
4. Loge, J. P.., Lange, R. D. and Moore, C. V. (1958). Characterization of the anaemia associated with chronic renal insufficiency. *Am. J. Med.*, **24**, 4–18
5. Caro, J., Brown, S., Miller, O., Murray, T. and Erslev, A. J. (1979). Erythropoietin levels in uremic nephric and anephric patients. *J. Lab. Clin. Med.*, **93**, 449–58
6. Mehls, O., Eberhard, R., Kerusser, W. and Krempien, B. (1980). Renal osteodystrophy in uremic children. *Clin. Endocrinol. Metab.*, **9**, 151–76
7. Norman, M. E., Mayur, A. T. and Borden, S. I. V. (1980). Early diagnosis of juvenile renal osteodystrophy. *J. Pediatr.*, **97**, 226
8. Blockey, N. J., Murphy, A. V. and Mocan, H. (1986). Management of rachitic deformities in children with chronic renal failure. *J. Bone Joint Surg.*, **68**, 791
9. Kleinknecht, C., Broyer, M. and Gagnadoux, M. (1980). Growth in children treated with long term dialysis. In Hamburger, J., Crosnier, J., Grunfeld, J. P. *et al.* (eds.), *Advances in Nephrology*. Vol. 19. (Chicago: Year Book Medical Publisher)
10. Salusky, I. B., Fine, R. N., Nelson, P., Blumenkranty, M. J. and Kepple, J. D. (1983). Nutritional status of children undergoing continuous ambulatory peritoneal dialysis. *Am. J. Clin. Nutr.*, **38**, 599–611
11. Combined Report on Regular Dialysis and Transplantation of children in Europe. (1979–1984). Published by Balliere Tindall, Eastbourne, and the Council of the European Dialysis and Transplant Association – European Renal Association, offered by Hospal Ltd., Basel
12. Harmon, W. E., Meyer, A. and Grupe, W. E. (1982). Substitution of a percutaneous vascular access for repeated haemodialysis in children. In Bulla, M. (ed.), *Renal Insufficiency in Children*. p. 173. (Berlin, Heidelberg, New York: Springer-Verlag)
13. Popovich, R. P., Moncrief, J. W. and Decherd, J. B. (1976). The definition of a novel portable/wearable equilibrium peritoneal dialysis technique. *Abst. Trans. Am. Soc. Artif. Intern. Organs*, **5**, 64
14. Persijh, G. G., Cohen, B. and Lansbergen, Q. (1982). Effect of HLA-A and HLA-B matching in survival of grafts and recipients after renal transplantation. *N. Engl. J. Med.*, **307**, 905
15. Opelz, G. and Terasaki, P. I. (1982). International study of histocompatibility in renal transplantation. *Transplantation*, **33**, 81
16. Fuller, T. C., Delmonico, F. L. and Cosini, A. B. (1978). Impact of blood transfusion on renal transplantation. *Ann. Surg.*, **187**, 211
17. Burke, J. R., Counahan, A. J. W. and Hilson, M. N. (1979). Serial quantitative imaging with ^{99m}Tc-DTPA in pediatric renal transplantation. *Clin. Nephrol.*, **12**, 174
18. Malekzaden, M., Grushkin, C. M. and Stanley, P. (1987). Renal artery stenosis in pediatric transplant recipients. *Pediatr. Nephrol.*, **1**, 22–9
19. Lewis, E. J. (1982), Recurrent focal sclerosis after renal transplantation. *Kidney Int.*, **22**, 315

20. Keenan, M. (1983). An investigation of the attitudes of patients, parents and staff to the treatment of chronic renal failure in children. Dissertation for degree of Master of Applied Science in Clinical Psychology, University of Glasgow
21. James, H. (1986). Attitudes towards illness and treatment in children with chronic renal failure: type of treatment, depression in parent and direct versus indirect measures of attitudes. Thesis for degree of MA Social Sciences in Psychology, University of Glasgow

3

SEXUAL AND ENDOCRINE FUNCTION IN URAEMIA

N. MUIRHEAD

INTRODUCTION

The kidney has long been recognized as a key organ in relation to endocrine function, both as a target site for hormones and as a major site of hormone metabolism. More recently the kidney has been found to possess a number of unique endocrine and paracrine activities in its own right. It is, therefore, no surprise that renal failure should be associated with such a wide variety of endocrine dysfunctions.

Hormone concentrations in chronic renal failure may be increased, decreased or normal. Disordered endocrine function may be related to these abnormal hormone concentrations or to abnormalities in peripheral hormone activity induced by renal failure. The principal endocrine abnormalities encountered in chronic renal failure are listed in Table 3.1.

Increased hormone concentrations

The serum concentrations of many hormones are increased in patients with chronic renal failure. This does not necessarily translate into disordered hormone function for a variety of reasons. Since the kidney is a major site of hormone metabolism, increases in hormone concentrations may in some cases result merely from impaired metabolic clearance rather than altered endocrine function. For example, the

TABLE 3.1 Endocrine abnormalities in chronic renal failure. See appropriate sections of text for details

Hormone	*Blood level*	*Mechanism(s)*
Insulin	increased	impaired catabolism; immunoheterogeneity
Glucagon	increased	impaired catabolism; immunoheterogeneity
Growth hormone	increased	impaired catabolism; immunoheterogeneity
Calcitonin	increased	impaired catabolism; immunoheterogeneity
Prolactin	increased	impaired catabolism; immunoheterogeneity increased secretion
PTH	increased	impaired catabolism; immunoheterogeneity; increased secretion; peripheral resistance
LH/FSH	increased	increased secretion
Erythropoietin	decreased	decreased renal secretion
$1,25(OH)_2D_3$	decreased	decreased renal secretion
Sex steroids	decreased	impaired testicular/ovarian function
Triiodothyronine	decreased	impaired peripheral conversion of T_4

kidney normally accounts for around one third of the metabolic clearance of insulin[1], glucagon[2] and somatostatin[3] and two thirds that of proinsulin[1], parathyroid hormone (PTH)[4], calcitonin[5], growth hormone[6] and prolactin[7]. Thus, increases in the serum concentrations of these hormones in chronic renal failure are at least partly explained by failure of renal metabolism.

Hormone assay methods may not invariably help to determine whether elevations in concentrations of peptide hormones, in particular, are in any way reflective of disordered endocrine function. It is known, for example, that serum PTH concentrations are elevated from an early stage in the course of chronic renal failure[8]. Much of the elevation in PTH is, however, due to the accumulation of fragments of varying length from the carboxy-terminal region of the hormone[9].

These fragments have no biological activity so that the measured PTH concentration does not accurately reflect the extent of parathyroid overactivity unless an assay directed at the biologically active amino-terminal region of the hormone is used[10]. In the case of PTH, the situation is further complicated by the fact that PTH secretion is truly increased[9,11], as well as PTH accumulating for the reasons outlined above.

Interpretation of serum insulin and glucagon concentrations in chronic renal failure is subject to similar problems. Proinsulin and C-peptide are substantially cleared by the kidney[1] and so tend to be disproportionately elevated in chronic renal failure[12]. High serum C-peptide concentration in particular may be misleading since it could lead to an erroneous diagnosis of adequate pancreatic β-cell reserve function in diabetic patients with renal failure. Additionally, high proinsulin and C-peptide could lead to a mistaken diagnosis of β-cell tumour in uraemic patients with hypoglycaemia. In the case of glucagon, the hormone responsible for increased circulating immunoreactive glucagon is most probably a biologically inactive glucagon precursor[13]. The concentrations of biologically active glucagon in renal failure and the responses to appropriate stimulatory or suppressive stimuli are reported to be normal in renal failure[14].

Some hormones are, however, truly secreted in increased amounts in renal failure. Examples include PTH[9,11], aldosterone[15] and atrial natriuretic peptide[16]. Increased secretion of these hormones is in many cases an adaptive measure aimed at maintaining the ability of the kidney to control sodium/water/calcium homeostasis.

Decreased hormone concentrations

The serum concentrations of a wide variety of hormones are reduced in renal failure. Hormone concentrations may be reduced because of impaired production by the kidney or other endocrine organs or impaired activation of or conversion to active hormones by peripheral tissues.

The kidney is the major site of synthesis of both erythropoietin and 1,25 dihydroxycholecalciferol (1,25$(OH)_2D_3$). Serum concentrations of erythropoietin are inappropriately low in the face of the anaemia of chronic renal failure and correlate with glomerular filtration rate (GFR)[17–19]. This suggests that failure of renal synthesis and/or release of erythropoietin is of importance in the pathogenesis of uraemic anaemia. Similarly, serum concentrations of $1,25(OH)_2D_3$ are low in renal failure as a result of impaired renal biosynthesis[20]. Lack of this hormonal form of vitamin D is of key importance in the development of metabolic bone disease in chronic renal failure.

The other major hormones whose serum concentrations tend to be low in renal failure are gonadal steroids and triiodothyronine (T_3). The reduced sex steroid concentrations result largely from reduced testicular[21] or ovarian[22] synthesis, though impaired tissue conversion to active metabolites may contribute to the consequent clinical features. Thyroid hormone concentrations are widely variable and difficult to interpret in renal failure. The one consistent finding is that T_3 is low or low–normal[23,24] in CRF as a result of impaired peripheral deiodination of thyroxine to T_3[25]. There remains considerable doubt as to the clinical significance of low T_3 in CRF and the need, if any, for treatment.

Altered hormone effect

For some hormones not only may their serum concentrations be altered but there is also an alteration in peripheral tissue sensitivity to the hormone that contributes to clinical endocrine dysfunction. Examples include PTH[11,26], atrial natriuretic peptide[27] and insulin[28]. Peripheral tissue sensitivity to these hormones is depressed in CRF and this is thought to contribute to their overproduction.

SPECIFIC ENDOCRINE DYSFUNCTION IN CHRONIC RENAL FAILURE

Thyroid function

As mentioned above, disturbances in thyroid function have been widely reported in patients with CRF. Most reports suggest that patients with CRF have at least laboratory evidence for hypothyroidism[23,24,29]. Equally there is no doubt that many of the symptoms associated with CRF – anaemia, cold intolerance, dry skin – are somewhat reminiscent of hypothyroidism. However, the few systematic clinical studies performed agree that there is no clinical evidence of hypothyroidism in patients with CRF[24]. The interpretation of thyroid function tests and diagnosis of true hypothyroidism are therefore fraught with difficulties in CRF.

The patterns of abnormalities in thyroid function tests in CRF are summarized in Table 3.2. The most consistently reported abnormality is the presence of a low or low–normal total T_3 in the presence of a normal total thyroxine (T_4)[23,24,30]. Direct measurement of free T_3 shows that this is also low suggesting that loss of T_3 is not due purely to alterations in thyroid hormone binding as evidenced by low free T_3 index (FT_3I)[31]. The most reasonable explanation for low total and free T_3 in CRF is that there is decreased peripheral conversion of T_4 to T_3 with shunting of T_4 metabolism to production of the metabolically inactive reverse T_3 (RT_3)[25,32]. It has been suggested that this reduced T_3 production may actually be an adaptive measure aimed at diminishing thyroid hormone-related catabolism in patients with severe non-thyroid disease such as CRF[32].

As mentioned earlier, there is no clinical evidence that CRF patients with these abnormalities of thyroid hormones are actually hypothyroid[24]. Indeed treatment with either T_4 or T_3 has no measurable

TABLE 3.2 Thyroid function tests in chronic renal failure. See text for detailed explanation

Test	*Result*	*Comment*
Total T_4	normal/low normal	may fall in long-term dialysis
Free T_4	normal (↑% total)	may ↑ transiently during dialysis (heparin effect)
Total T_3	low/low normal	due to ↓ conversion $T_4 \rightarrow T_3$
Free T_3	decreased (normal or ↑% total)	
RT_3	normal	contrasts with 'euthyroid sick' in which RT_3 is high
TSH	normal	best indicator of hypothyroidism
TRH test	variable TSH response	not reliable as thyroid function test in CRF

impact on symptoms[33]. These abnormalities can make the diagnosis of true hypothyroidism difficult. It has been suggested that serum TSH concentration is the most reliable diagnostic test for secondary hypothyroidism in patients with CRF[34].

The response to TRH stimulation in patients with CRF may also be abnormal. There remains some controversy on this point since both blunted and exaggerated responses of TSH to TRH stimulation have been reported in CRF. Most reports agree that release of T_3 from the thyroid during TRH stimulation is subnormal, irrespective of the TSH response[25,29]. This has been taken to imply that there is abnormal sensitivity of the hypothalamic-pituitary-thyroid axis in CRF. Thus the normal TSH concentrations found in CRF in the face of often profound decreases in free T_3, suggest hypersensitivity to feedback inhibition, most probably at the hypothalamic level.

The use of thyroid hormone concentrations to diagnose hypothyroidism may therefore be difficult in CRF. Characteristically, total and free T_3 are low while total T_4 is normal. Total RT_3 is normal in CRF in contrast to the 'euthyroid sick syndrome' in which total and free RT_3 are high. Serum TSH is normal in euthyroid patients with CRF and may offer the single best indicator of hypothyroidism in uraemic subjects.

In summary, there are profound alterations in serum concentration of thyroid hormones in uraemia which confuse the diagnosis of hypothyroidism. These abnormalities are subtly different from the 'euthyroid sick syndrome' and may well represent a true adaptation to the reduced metabolic demand of uraemia.

Adrenocortical steroids

Cortisol

In CRF serum concentrations of both free and conjugated 17-hydroxycorticosteroids (17-OHCS) are elevated as a result of impaired renal excretion[35,36]. Clearance of cortisol from the serum is also delayed, perhaps as a result of reduced hepatic metabolism related in some way to uraemia[37,38]. Haemodialysis, with its rapid haemodynamic changes, might be expected to cause alterations in adrenocortical function and has therefore been the topic of considerable interest.

Early studies suggested that plasma cortisol levels fell initially during a haemodialysis session, due to removal of cortisol by dialysis, and rebounded towards the end of haemodialysis so that cortisol levels were in fact elevated at the end of a dialysis session[39,40]. More recent studies have indicated that there is no significant removal of cortisol by haemodialysis as would be anticipated from the fact that cortisol is largely protein bound[38,41]. Indeed it now appears that plasma cortisol concentrations are, if anything, elevated at the start of haemodialysis and remain so during the procedure[37].

Evaluation of the pattern of cortisol secretion in haemodialysis patients reveals that the normal circadian rhythm is maintained on both dialysis and non-dialysis days, though plasma cortisol tends to be higher on dialysis days[37]. Although the elevated plasma cortisols in haemodialysis patients can, in part, be explained by impaired metabolic clearance, there is additional evidence for increased secretion. The most likely explanation for increased secretion of cortisol is an alteration of hypothalamic-pituitary sensitivity to feedback inhibition by cortisol[37,42].

It would be expected that, if the hypothalamic-pituitary-adrenal axis were functioning normally in CRF, the modest increases in plasma cortisol reported by most investigators would be accompanied by a reduction in serum adrenocorticotrophin (ACTH) concentrations. In fact ACTH concentrations are modestly elevated in patients with CRF[43,44]. Serum concentrations of the other secretory products of pituitary corticotrophs (lipotropins (LPH), β-endorphins) are considerably elevated in CRF[44]. Both ACTH and β-LPH are derived from intrapituitary cleavage of a common precursor molecule and are secreted simultaneously. The differential effects of CRF on their serum concentrations are due to a difference in metabolic clearance. Normally the metabolic clearance of β-LPH exceeds that of ACTH[45] but the situation is reversed in CRF[44].

Since the metabolic clearance of ACTH is unaltered by CRF the combination of elevated ACTH and plasma cortisol reflects disordered feedback control of pituitary function. Several studies have indicated that in CRF plasma cortisol fails to suppress normally in response to dexamethasone[42,43], suggesting that an elevation in the set point of negative feedback control may underly the alterations in hypothalamic-pituitary-adrenocortical axis function. Similar abnormalities in the cortisol response to dexamethasone suppression have been reported in protein-calorie malnutrition.

Failure of normal ACTH response to appropriate stimuli is suggested by the finding of blunted ACTH response to insulin-induced hypoglycaemia and metyrapone in CRF[43,46]. Thus feedback regulation of ACTH at the hypothalamic and pituitary level may also be abnormal.

At the clinical level some of the symptoms seen in CRF, such as weakness, hypotension and pigmentation, are reminiscent of symptoms of hypoadrenalism. However, as noted above, the plasma concentration of adrenocortical steroids are increased in CRF. Hypoadrenalism is therefore an unlikely explanation of weakness and hypotension in CRF. Serum concentrations of melanocyte stimulating hormone (β-MSH), a breakdown product of β-LPH, are elevated in CRF and may contribute to uraemic pigmentation[47].

Of more relevance is the ability to distinguish the abnormalities of ACTH and cortisol in CRF from a diagnosis of pituitary-dependent Cushing's syndrome. In CRF the normal circadian rhythm of cortisol secretion is maintained and although the response to dexamethasone suppression in CRF is incomplete, there is some suppression, in contrast to the failure of cortisol suppression by dexamethasone in true pituitary-driven Cushing's syndrome[42].

Aldosterone

Aldosterone is an adrenocortical steroid intimately involved in the control of urinary sodium excretion. Its secretion is largely unrelated to the activity of ACTH. Since in CRF there are profound alterations in the handling of sodium and water, it is not surprising that aldosterone secretion is also altered in CRF.

Plasma aldosterone concentrations are generally elevated in CRF[48]. This may be seen as an adaptive measure aimed at preventing sodium wasting. Lack of mineralocorticoid activity in CRF is associated with natriuresis and hyperkalaemia. This condition (hyporeninaemic-hypoaldosteronism) is being recognized with increasing frequency, particularly in diabetics with CRF[49]. It is characterized by the development of a hyperkalaemic metabolic acidosis (Type IV renal tubular acidosis). Effective therapy is possible with mineralocorticoid replacement[50]. It is probable that aldosterone hypersecretion in CRF helps counterbalance this tendency to natriuresis, probably due to increased atrial natriuretic factor (ANF)[15]. In late CRF and dialysis patients, the anti-natriuretic effect of aldosterone is less important since at that stage frank sodium retention occurs and natriuretic influences therefore predominate[51,52].

The role of aldosterone in patients on haemodialysis is uncertain. Plasma aldosterone in such patients is increased and responds normally to changes in serum potassium in particular[48,53]. It seems probable that aldosterone has actions in many extra-renal sites and may therefore defend against hyperkalaemia by permitting potassium entry into cells generally. Thus, the rise in plasma aldosterone seen in CRF patients in response to hyperkalaemia may limit the rise in serum potassium.

Erythropoietin

Although it would be naive to assume that lack of erythropoietin (EPO) is the sole cause of the anaemia of CRF, there now seems little doubt that it is a major contributor[16,17,54]. A number of factors are responsible for anaemia affecting up to 98% of haemodialysis patients (Table 3.3).

EPO is a glycoprotein hormone that is secreted by the kidneys in response to the stimulus of tissue hypoxia. It is likely that the liver also can secrete small amounts of EPO, although the regulatory factors and potential biological role of hepatic EPO secretion are at present unknown. Serum EPO concentrations, whether measured by bioassay or radioimmunoassay techniques, are consistently within the normal range for non-anaemic adults in CRF[16,17,54]. This most probably represents hepatic EPO secretion. In non-uraemic adults with comparable degrees of anaemia, serum EPO concentrations are greatly elevated[55]. Thus the normal EPO concentrations seen in CRF represent a severe failure of EPO secretion in response to a normally powerful stimulus.

Experimental studies of sheep EPO on a variety of animal models of CRF have shown that the accompanying anaemia can be greatly improved. Preliminary studies of a recombinant human EPO (r-HuEPO)

TABLE 3.3 Factors contributing to anaemia in chronic renal failure. Erythropoietin and blood loss from dialysis and iatrogenic causes are the most significant

(1)	Erythropoietin deficiency
(2)	Haemolysis – intravascular ?related to PTH
(3)	Blood loss gastrointestinal dialyser/blood lines iatrogenic, i.e. routine 'tests'
(4)	Deficiency of haematinics Fe – dietary folic acid – loss via dialyser, dietary B_{12} – loss via dialyser, diet

in patients with CRF have shown a similar beneficial response[56,57]. The availability of biosynthetic human EPO to treat the anaemia of CRF represents a major therapeutic advance. There is no doubt that anaemia is a major cause of morbidity in CRF. Around 35% of patients on haemodialysis require frequent blood transfusions to maintain haemoglobin. A further 30% of haemodialysis patients require periodic blood transfusions.

Enthusiasm for blood transfusion in uraemic patients has waxed and waned over the years. In the 1960s and early 1970s, blood transfusion was considered undesirable because of the risk of transmitting infections such as hepatitis B and the fear that allosensitization would reduce the chance of successful renal transplantation. From the mid-1970s onwards, the somewhat paradoxical beneficial effects of blood transfusion in improving renal transplant survival have encouraged a general relaxation of attitudes towards blood transfusion for dialysis patients and, in many instances, a policy of deliberate blood transfusion aimed at enhancing renal allograft survival. Effective screening for hepatitis B and the availability of an effective vaccine have also greatly reduced the risks of transmission of serum hepatitis. Recently the beneficial effects of transfusion on transplant survival have again been questioned, while there is renewed fear of transmission of non-A, non-B hepatitis and especially AIDS via blood transfusion. Increasing concern amongst both patients and physicians has increased the pressure to find alternatives to blood transfusion for therapy of anaemia in CRF.

Haematinics and androgens do produce a limited improvement in haemoglobin concentration in patients with uraemia[58,59]. Preliminary studies of recombinant human EPO in patients with CRF on haemodialysis have shown that it is effective in raising haemoglobin with few side-effects if care is taken to titrate the dose of EPO to produce a slow, steady rise in haemoglobin[56,57,60]. It is likely that preparations of human EPO will be available in the near future to treat the anaemia of CRF and a wide range of other conditions.

Vitamin D endocrine system

PTH and 1,25(OH)$_2$D$_3$

A detailed discussion of the abnormalities in calcium metabolism that result from altered secretion of these hormones in CRF is beyond the scope of this chapter. A brief discussion of the relevant pathophysiological principles follows.

From an early stage in the development of CRF (GFR 60–80 ml/min), there is a detectable rise in serum PTH concentrations[11,61]. Some of this rise in PTH is the result of reduced metabolic clearance of the hormone by the kidneys, site of two thirds of normal degradation, but in addition it is clear that there is increased production of PTH, in response to subtle changes in serum calcium and phosphate concentrations.

The pathogenesis of this secondary hyperparathyroidism is still controversial though the two main theories – phosphate retention and vitamin D deficiency – are by no means mutually exclusive. The phosphate retention theory was espoused by Bricker and Slatopolsky[62] and is detailed in Figure 3.1. This theory suggests that there is a trade-off between the tendency to develop hyperphosphataemia as GFR declines and the need to maintain serum calcium within the normal range such that excess phosphate is excreted by the kidneys and serum calcium maintained only at the expense of a progressive rise in serum PTH concentrations.

The role of vitamin D deficiency in the pathogenesis of secondary hyperparathyroidism is suggested by the finding of defective skeletal

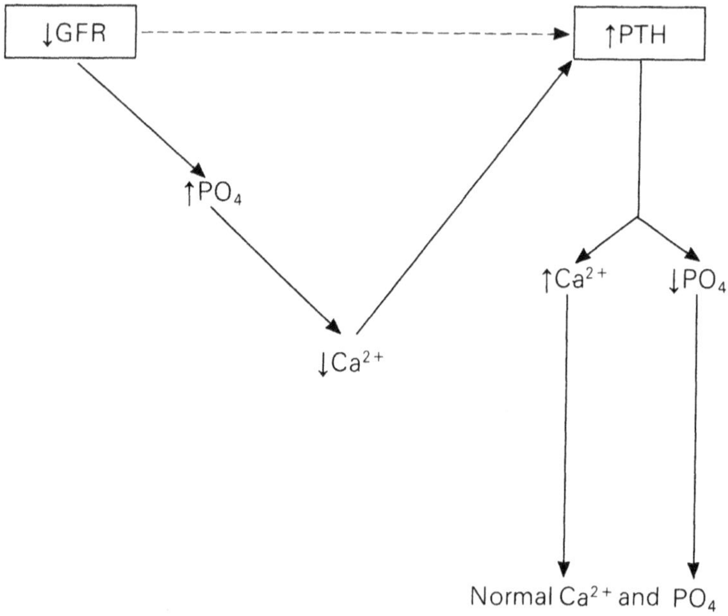

FIGURE 3.1 The phosphate retention theory. Pathogenesis of secondary hyperparathyroidism in CRF according to the phosphate retention theory of Bricker and Slatopolsky. Reduction in GFR is accompanied by a progressive rise in PTH with plasma Ca^{2+} and PO_4 remaining normal. The trade-off theory holds that progressive hyperparathyroidism is due to a reduction in Ca^{2+} induced by the rise in PO_4. PTH effect on the kidney restores Ca^{2+} and PO_4 to normal so that only the fall in GFR and rise in PTH remain detectable

mineralization in bone biopsies from patients with early CRF[63]. In addition, the most frequent abnormalities in serum calcium and phosphate in patients with early CRF is for both to be low, a pattern reminiscent of vitamin D deficiency. Serum concentrations of $1,25(OH)_2D_3$ are reported to be normal or even modestly increased in early CRF[64,65]. However, since these patients are typically mildly hypocalcaemic and hypophosphataemic, both of which should increase $1,25(OH)_2D_3$ levels, serum $1,25(OH)_2D_3$ is regarded as being inappropriately low and thus indicative of relative vitamin D deficiency.

As renal failure advances, serum PTH concentration rises progressively, though the contribution of circulating biologically inactive C-terminal fragments is more marked than the increase in intact hormone[66]. Thus measurement of PTH, by a method that recognizes predominantly C-terminal fragments, may give a false impression of the degree of parathyroid overactivity. At GFR <30 ml/min the capacity of the kidney to compensate for dietary phosphate intake, by increasing urinary phosphate, is overcome and frank hyperphosphataemia develops[62,67]. Since hyperphosphataemia is a powerful inhibitor of renal $1,25(OH)_2D_3$ production, this is also the stage at which levels of that hormone decline abruptly (Figure 3.2).

The terminal stages of CRF are therefore characterized by profoundly low serum concentrations of $1,25(OH)_2D_3$ and very high concentrations of PTH accompanied by marked hypocalcaemia and hyperphosphataemia. Once regular dialysis therapy is initiated the situation may change again. The majority of patients are dialysed against a dialysate that is high in calcium relative to the patient. Dialysis also removes phosphate. Thus haemodialysis in particular favours modest suppression of secondary hyperparathyroidism[68]. Serum concentrations of $1,25(OH)_2D_3$ are unaffected by dialysis.

The clinical consequences of these disorders of PTH and $1,25(OH)_2D_3$ metabolism are significant. The progressive rise in PTH during the often prolonged course of uraemia results in a metabolic bone disease (osteitis fibrosa) on which is superimposed a mineralization defect due to relative vitamin D deficiency[69]. The main symptoms are bone pain, spontaneous fractures, skeletal deformity and pruritus. While none of these symptoms are life-threatening, they do represent a considerable morbidity for individual patients.

A small number of patients with overt secondary hyperparathyroidism may go on to develop frank hypercalcaemia, either spontaneously or in response to small amounts of exogenous $1,25(OH)_2D_3$[70]. These patients have been, in the past, labelled as having tertiary hyperparathyroidism, since PTH failed to suppress in such patients in response to a calcium infusion[71]. Recent studies utilizing an N-terminal specific PTH assay suggest that PTH sensitivity to the stimulus of hypercalcaemia is maintained in CRF but that the threshold for PTH secretion may be increased[10]. Thus PTH secretion in hypercalcaemic dialysis patients persists, despite the fact that a further increase in serum calcium with a calcium infusion can induce

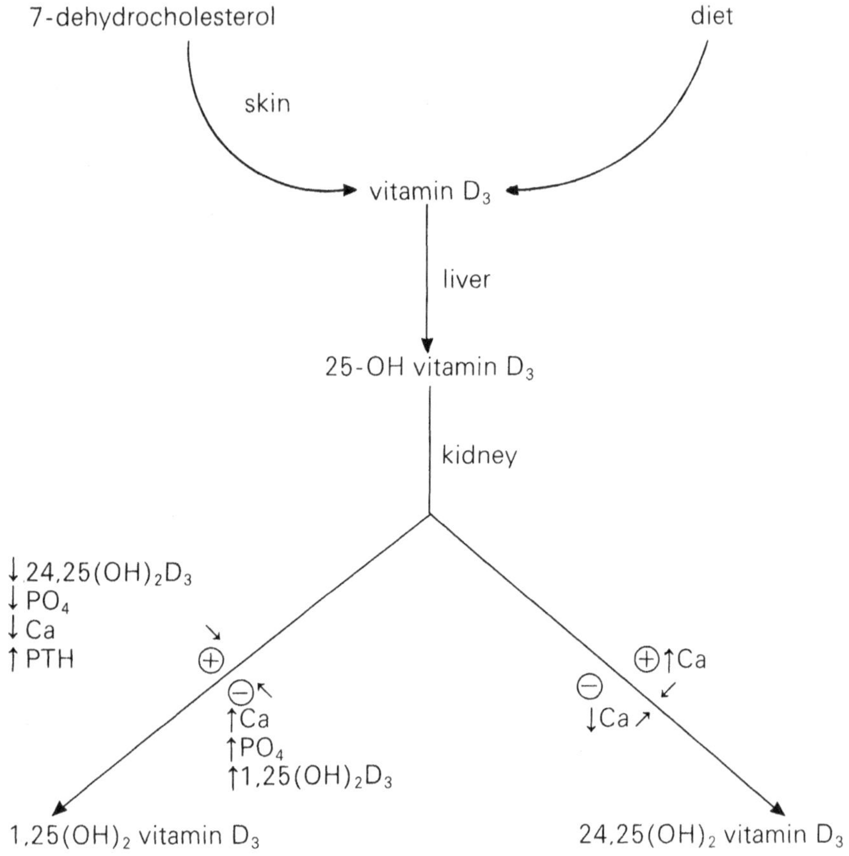

FIGURE 3.2 Metabolism of vitamin D_3. Vitamin D_3 is obtained via the diet and from photoconversion of 7-dehydrocholesterol in sun-exposed skin. Initial hydroxylation occurs in the liver and final hydroxylation in the kidney. In vitamin D replete individuals 24,25$(OH)_2$ vitamin D_3 is the predominant product of renal vitamin D metabolism. It has no critical biological actions in man. Renal production of 1,25$(OH)_2$ vitamin D_3 is strictly regulated

an appropriate fall in serum PTH[10]. This mechanism may also at least partly explain the transient hypercalcaemia that occurs in up to a third of patients following successful renal transplantation[72,73].

For the majority of patients with CRF, metabolic bone disease may be managed by giving a small replacement dose of $1,25(OH)_2D_3$ (0.25–0.5 μg) by mouth, along with control of serum phosphate with oral phosphate binders such as aluminium hydroxide and calcium supplementation as required. Such a regimen will lead to healing of metabolic bone disease in over 70% of cases[74]. A small proportion of patients with advanced hyperparathyroid bone disease may require parathyroidectomy in order to achieve clinical control of bone disease. Prophylactic use of $1,25(OH)_2D_3$ in patients with CRF, prior to dialysis, is now an established therapy.

Parathyroid hormone as a uraemic toxin

Although the principal effects of PTH excess in uraemia are on calcium and phosphate metabolism there has been considerable speculation that PTH is a more general uraemic toxin[75]. Secondary hyperparathyroidism has been implicated as a cause of uraemic neuropathy, sexual dysfunction, uraemic cardiomyopathy, anaemia and uraemic bleeding.

PTH has been implicated as a cause of uraemic neuropathy[76]. The mechanism is uncertain but would most probably involve generalized effects on cellular calcium metabolism induced directly or indirectly by PTH. There is clear evidence that PTH causes calcium ingress into a wide variety of mammalial cell types from both *in vitro* and *in vivo* experiments[77]. The relationship between these observations and clinical disorders in chronic renal failure attributable to PTH as a uraemic toxin remain speculative. Clinical and experimental studies have suggested a link between PTH concentrations in CRF and alterations in both motor nerve conduction and electroencephalographic (EEG) abnormalities[76,78]. Parathyroidectomy has been reported to improve impaired nerve conduction and restore the EEG to normal[76,78].

It has been suggested that PTH may influence the development of uraemic hypogonadism[75,79]. An inverse relationship between PTH and testosterone has been reported in CRF, with improvement in plasma testosterone following reduction in PTH, irrespective of any changes in LH or FSH.

The view that PTH may act as a cardiac toxin in uraemia has

received considerable attention[75,80]. Clinical and experimental studies have suggested a negative inotropic effect of PTH[80], while other recent studies have failed to demonstrate any consistent effect of PTH on cardiac function[81]. Whether PTH acts as a cardiac toxin through direct effects on myocardial cell calcium metabolism or indirectly via autonomic nervous or hormonal control of cardiac function is unknown. Abnormal autonomic function, evidenced by reduced pressor response to noradrenaline, is common in CRF[81]. PTH can be shown to block the pressor effects of both noradrenaline and angiotension II in rats, an effect that is blocked by indomethacin, a prostaglandin synthetase inhibitor[81,82]. It is therefore suggested that the effects of PTH on modulating response to noradrenaline and angiotensin II in uraemia are mediated through increased prostaglandin production. One recent study has implied a direct relationship between serum PTH concentrations and pressor response to noradrenaline in patients with CRF[81]. The precise relationship, if any, of secondary hyperparathyroidism to uraemic cardiomyopathy remains uncertain at the present time.

The relationship between PTH and the anaemia of CRF is complex. PTH has been reported to increase the osmotic fragility of human red blood cells (RBCs) *in vitro* and hence enhances haemolysis[83]. The mechanism of this effect is felt to be an increase in RBC calcium content which in turn leads to rigidity of the RBC membrane, decreased deformability and thus a tendency to haemolysis in both blood and spleen[84]. There is some circumstantial evidence that PTH may be one factor determining the osmotic fragility of RBCs in patients with CRF and hence may contribute to anaemia via increased haemolysis[84]. Of further importance is the role of hyperparathyroidism on bone marrow function. At one extreme, excessive marrow fibrosis induced by severe secondary hyperparathyroidism can certainly limit erythropoiesis, resulting in a form of secondary myelofibrosis[85]. More controversial is the concept that PTH may have an active role in suppressing erythropoiesis. This view has been challenged by recent *in vitro* studies which demonstrate that although uraemic serum inhibits erythropoiesis, this inhibitor is not PTH[86]. The most likely effects of PTH on anaemia in CRF would appear therefore to reside in production of haemolysis and secondary myelofibrosis.

A possible role for PTH in causing the decreased platelet function observed in uraemia has been suggested[87]. PTH has been shown to inhibit platelet aggregation *in vitro*, using concentrations similar to those achieved in uraemic plasma[87]. Clinical studies have failed to show any consistent relationship between PTH and platelet function[88].

In summary, PTH excess has been implicated as a uraemic toxin with wide ranging clinical manifestations. Despite the body of theoretical and circumstantial evidence in support of this view, the concept of PTH as a key uraemic toxin remains unproven. Further studies, currently in progress, will perhaps clarify this issue.

Atrial natriuretic peptide

The existence of a natriuretic hormone was suspected for many years. Recently, a series of peptides with natriuretic, diuretic and vasodilatory properties has been isolated from atrial myocytes in a number of species including man[89,90]. Several of these peptides have now been sequenced and synthesized and their use in a variety of experimental and clinical circumstances has led to an improved understanding of the complexities of control of intraglomerular haemodynamics and glomerular filtration.

The major stimulus to secretion of atrial natriuretic peptide (ANP) is an increase in atrial pressure, whether by saline loading, balloon dilatation or a high sodium diet[91,92]. The secretory response to infusion of ADH, angiotensin II, DOCA or phenylephrine suggests that ANP secretion is closely related to volume status. Actual or perceived volume expansion leads to increased ANP secretion in an effort to restore blood volume to normal.

The main actions of ANP on the kidney are to increase GFR and induce natriuresis[93]. It is likely that the increase in GFR occurs as a result of alterations in intraglomerular haemodynamics. The natriuresis occurs partly as a result of the increase in GFR but there also appears to be a direct effect of ANP on sodium handling by medullary collecting ducts[94].

In patients with CRF there is clear evidence for enhanced ANP secretion[16]. This increase is viewed by many investigators as an adaptive measure to the loss in nephron mass which would otherwise lead to sodium and water retention. It seems likely that hypersecretion of

ANP permits the maintenance of sodium homeostasis until an advanced stage of CRF. Indeed clinical sodium overload is rare in CRF at GFR >5 ml/min.

ANP concentration is elevated in haemodialysis patients[16]. The clinical relevance of this in unknown, though it may contribute to hypertension through its ability to cause peripheral vasoconstriction under conditions of volume expansion.

Carbohydrate metabolism

Carbohydrate intolerance ('uraemic pseudodiabetes') is found in over 50% of patients with end-stage renal disease[95]. Fasting blood sugar in such patients is usually normal, while oral or i.v. glucose tolerance tests show a diabetic response[96,97]. This condition clearly makes the the diagnosis of true diabetes difficult in CRF. Of more practical relevance is the question of whether the abnormalities in carbohydrate metabolism may be responsible for the hyperlipidaemia and atherosclerosis that frequently accompany CRF[98].

Despite clear glucose intolerance in CRF, fasting plasma insulin is uniformly increased in non-diabetics with CRF[95,99]. The insulin response to oral or i.v. glucose is variable in uraemia. The early insulin response to an oral glucose tolerance test (GTT) has been reported to be normal or increased in uraemia[97]. In contrast, the early insulin response to i.v. glucose has been reported to be reduced, normal or exaggerated in CRF[95,97,100], while there is general agreement that hyperinsulinaemia persists during the latter part of both i.v. and oral GTTs in uraemic patients[95,100]. The conflicting data may in part reflect the population under study. Initiation of adequate haemodialysis has been reported to restore the GTT and insulin responses to normal[101].

The aetiology of hyperinsulinaemia in CRF is due in part to reduced degradation of insulin by the kidneys[1]. Under normal circumstances around one third of insulin is cleared by the kidney, the remainder by the liver and skeletal muscle[1,102]. Although impaired renal clearance is mainly responsible for hyperinsulinaemia in CRF, reduced extrarenal clearance has also been reported. The role of altered secretion rates of insulin in the production of uraemic hyperinsulinaemia remains unclear.

In diabetics with renal failure progressive uraemia is characterized by reduced insulin requirements and improvement in blood sugar control[103]. Ketoacidosis is rare in diabetics with end-stage renal failure[103,104]. The improvements in blood glucose control are due in part to reduced renal clearance of insulin, though reduced caloric intake (due to anorexia) and impaired glycogenolysis may also contribute[103]. Spontaneous hypoglycaemia occurs in both diabetics and non-diabetics with CRF. In diabetics the main precipitating factors are likely to be impaired glycogenolysis and prolonged insulin activity with reduced renal and hepatic gluconeogenesis playing perhaps a minor role. Profound hypoglycaemia, especially fasting, is seen on occasion in non-diabetic uraemic subjects[105,106]. The exact mechanism is obscure but a number of factors may contribute. Firstly systemic acidosis has been shown to impair hepatic gluconeogenesis which might therefore be expected to produce fasting hypoglycaemia[107]. Propranolol has been implicated in uraemic hypoglycaemia by causing impairment of hepatic glycogenolysis[108]. Deficiency of substrates for hepatic gluconeogenesis, specifically alanine, has also been suggested as a possible cause of uraemic hypoglycaemia[106]. In this context, nutritional deprivation has been associated with uraemic hypoglycaemia, with improvement in symptoms noted after nutrition improved.

The observation of normal fasting blood sugar in association with fasting hyperinsulinaemia has led to the suggestion that there is impaired tissue responsiveness to insulin in uraemia. There is now considerable evidence in support of this theory, especially in relation to impaired responsiveness of skeletal muscle to insulin[109,110]. The finding of impaired tissue responsiveness to exogenous insulin in CRF suggests that immunoheterogeneity of insulin in CRF is unlikely to be due to the circulation of an abnormal insulin.

Impaired tissue responsiveness may be due to impaired binding of insulin to tissue receptors or alterations in postreceptor events. Studies of insulin interaction with receptors in CRF have yielded conflicting results with binding reported to be reduced, normal or increased depending on the tissue or animal species used and the presence/absence of dialysis therapy.

The role of postreceptor defects is similarly unclear. One recent study suggested that in skeletal muscle, glucose utilization was impaired in uraemic subjects due to a postreceptor defect in glucose metabolism[111]. This study was unable, however, to differentiate clearly between a postreceptor defect and altered insulin-receptor interaction. Since little is known about insulin binding to skeletal muscle receptors in CRF, the concept that tissue insulin resistance in uraemia is due primarily to altered postreceptor glucose metabolism remains unproven.

Improvement in glucose tolerance and tissue insulin responsiveness characteristically follow initiation of dialysis[99,112,113]. This suggests that dialysable factors are of importance in the pathogenesis of carbohydrate intolerance in uraemia. Such factors have yet to be identified.

A number of non-dialysable peptides are secreted in abnormal amounts in CRF and may therefore contribute to the abnormal glucose metabolism seen. Growth hormone (GH) levels are often raised in CRF but do not correlate with the degree of carbohydrate intolerance seen[95,114]. The major cause of GH excess is impaired degradation by the kidneys[6] though a paradoxical increase in secretion, due perhaps to protein-calorie malnutrition, has also been observed following glucose loading[115].

Hyperglucagonaemia is frequently observed in CRF[116,117]. As noted above, this is due in part to secretion of a biologically inactive glucagon precursor[117,118] and in part due to decreased renal elimination[10]. However, plasma levels of bioactive glucagon are also reportedly elevated in CRF and may therefore contribute to abnormal carbohydrate metabolism in CRF[117,118]. The relationship of GH or glucagon excess to carbohydrate intolerance in uraemia is unclear since the improvement in carbohydrate tolerance noted above after initiation of haemodialysis occurs without measurable alterations in bioactive GH or glucagon levels.

On a clinical level, abnormal carbohydrate tolerance in CRF may occasionally cause diagnostic confusion in patients with Type II diabetes and renal failure. The presence of hyperinsulinaemia and hypoglycaemia in CRF may lead to the erroneous diagnosis of an insulinoma. Measurement of insulin, C-peptide and glucagon during hypoglycaemia will usually allow insulinoma to be differentiated from uraemic hypoglycaemia.

Of more concern is the possible relationship between uraemic carbohydrate intolerance, hyperlipidaema and atheroma. Around 60% of patients with CRF are hyperlipidaemic, typically with hypertriglyceridaemia and normal or low total cholesterol[98,119,120]. The combination of hyperinsulinaemia, impaired tissue responsiveness to insulin and hypertriglyceridaemia seen in CRF is reminiscent of the situation in obesity and has led to the suggestion of a pathogenetic relationship between the carbohydrate and lipid abnormalities. Subsequent studies in man have shown that the triglyceride synthesis rate is diminished in CRF and that the principal mechanism of hypertriglyceridaemia is reduced assimilation of triglycerides by adipose tissue[121]. In addition, the relationship of hyperlipidaemia to both atheroma or progressive cardiovascular disease in CRF has recently been questioned[122]. It is therefore difficult to make a case for drug treatment of uraemic hyperlipidaemia.

Gastrin

A host of gastroduodenal symptoms including anorexia, nausea, vomiting, gastritis and peptic ulcer (PU) are reported in excess in CRF[123]. Elevation of the serum gastrin concentration has been reported in uraemia[124] and may be a cause of peptic ulceration and other gastrointestinal symptoms in such patients. A number of recent reports have indicated that, in fact, gastric acid production is typically low in CRF, despite hypergastrinaemia, due to impaired parietal cell function[125,126]. A recent study demonstrated inverse relationships between serum gastrin concentrations and both the gastric acid secretory response to pentagastrin and the occurrence of gastroduodenal erosions at endoscopy[126]. It has thus been suggested that hypergastrinaemia in CRF is a compensatory response to diminished parietal cell function. It is possible that hypergastrinaemia may in fact protect against gastric erosion by enhancing gastric motility and hence reducing biliary reflux.

The idea that PU is much commoner in patients with CRF has recently been challenged[127]. The majority of studies which suggested an increased risk of PU in uraemia involved small numbers of patients and thus inevitably included some selection bias. A recent survey of almost 250 dialysis patients surveyed as part of a pre-renal transplant evaluation reported a 11.2% prevalence of PU at endoscopy[127]. This compares with an estimated 10–14% prevalence of chronic PU in asymptomatic Western patients. It thus seems probable that the prevalence of PU in uraemia is not increased as was previously suspected.

SEXUAL DYSFUNCTION IN CHRONIC RENAL FAILURE

Introduction

There is no doubt that profound disturbances in sexual function are an almost invariable consequence of chronic renal failure[128]. Equally there is no doubt that the serum concentrations, secretion rates and metabolism of sex hormones are variably deranged in chronic renal failure. What remains uncertain is the extent to which measurable alterations in sex hormone levels or metabolism are responsible for disorders in sexual function in uraemia.

A variety of non-hormonal factors have been implicated in the pathogenesis of disordered sexual function in uraemia. These include vascular abnormalities, which affect erectile function in particular[129]; zinc deficiency, which has been implicated as a cause of secondary gonadal failure[130,131]; medications producing altered vascular or sex hormone function[132,133]; and finally, psychological factors[134]. In any given patient, more than one of these factors may be involved, irrespective of there being any alterations in sex hormone concentrations. This can lead to considerable difficulties in both diagnosis and therapy.

The most frequently reported abnormalities in sexual function in uraemia are lack of libido, impotence and infertility in men[135] and menstrual irregularities, loss of libido and infertility in women[22,136]. The incidence of disordered sexual function is reported to be 80% in uraemic men on haemodialysis. The reported incidence of disordered sexual function in uraemic women is much lower than in uraemic men. The problem is, however, considerably under-estimated; a recent review from Italy revealed that 80% of uraemic women in a number of centres reported disorders in sexual function[137]. It seems likely, therefore, that abnormal sexual function is an almost invariable accompaniment of chronic renal failure and affects uraemic men and women with equal frequency.

Although for ease of understanding, disorders in sex hormone metabolism will be discussed separately, there are many common themes in the pathogenesis of altered sex hormone function in uraemic men and women.

Sexual dysfunction in uraemic men

The main symptoms of sexual dysfunction in uraemic men are impotence, lack of libido and infertility. Such symptoms are rarely volunteered by patients unless specifically asked but may nevertheless be the source of a considerable degree of morbidity in terms of their effect on interpersonal relationships, self-esteem and self-image. While such considerations may seem trivial in the overall care of a patient who has a major medical illness (i.e. CRF) they are often of major importance to the patient and thus deserve an honest attempt on the part of the physician to understand the nature of the problem and, if possible, provide effective therapy. It is worth pointing out that not all uraemic impotence, for example, is due to untreatable factors vaguely related to renal failure. Drug-related or psychogenic impotence may be successfully treated by withdrawal of the offending drug or psychotherapy, while impotence related to vascular insufficiency can be treated by means of a penile implant.

Sex hormones in uraemic men

There is good evidence for functional impairment of the hypothalamic-pituitary-testicular axis in uraemic men. Sperm counts are low (or absent) with numerous sperm abnormal in terms of mobility and morphology[138,139]. This is reflected in abnormalities in testicular histology including reduced spermatogenesis, germinal cell aplasia and altered interstitial cell morphology[22,139]. The latter abnormality correlates with disordered interstitial cell function, i.e. reduced testosterone secretion. Plasma levels of total and free testosterone and of dihydrotestosterone are usually low in uraemia, both in the basal state and in response to the administration of human chorionic gonadotrophin (HCG)[21,140]. This has been taken to indicate functional impairment of testicular hormone biosynthesis and release. Haemodialysis produces a temporary increase in plasma testosterone levels, suggesting that 'uraemic toxins' may be important in the pathogenesis of testicular failure in uraemia[141]. However, recovery of testicular function sufficient to restore fertility in men on haemodialysis is very rare[142]. The site of the defect in testosterone biosynthesis is thought to be the reaction 17-hydroxypregnenolone→DHA (dehydroisoandrosterone) catalysed by the enzyme desmolase C17–20[143].

Most males with CRF have elevated luteinizing hormone (LH) levels due both to increased secretion and reduced metabolic clearance[21,139,143,144]. LH secretion rates are around 20% higher than in non-uraemic controls due to the relatively low plasma testosterone levels in uraemic men[144]. Serum levels of follicle stimulating hormone (FSH) are less often increased unless spermatogenesis is grossly deranged[139,143]. The correlation between FSH levels and spermatogenesis has prognostic value in predicting the potential for recovery of spermatogenesis following renal transplantation[142]. Where serum FSH is grossly elevated in CRF, spermatogenesis is usually so grossly abnormal that recovery cannot be expected with transplantation. In some uraemic patients low testosterone concentrations are accompanied by low LH levels, suggesting an abnormality of hypothalamic-pituitary function in addition to testicular failure[138,145]. The response of pituitary gonadotrophins to LHRH is reported to be normal in magnitude and duration in uraemic men, suggesting that synthesis, storage and release of FSH and LH are normal[138,144]. This does not exclude the possibility that abnormal feedback control could result in a resetting of LH secretion at lower than normal levels of testosterone[21,138,145]. In this context, long-term therapy with clomiphene in uraemic men will increase FSH and LH levels and restore testosterone secretion without necessarily improving spermatogenesis[146]. Further evidence that abnormal feedback control may be of more than passing importance is the observation that the restoration of normal spermatogenesis following successful renal transplantation is accompanied by a further increase in FSH levels[138].

The factor(s) that initiate these abnormalities in sex hormone function remain uncertain. That they are the major cause of sexual dysfunction in uraemic men is suggested by the partial or total reversal of the functional and hormonal disturbances after transplantation[136,138,142].

Sexual dysfunction in uraemic women

There are many similarities in the disturbances of sex hormone metabolism in uraemic women and men. Irregular menstruation and amenorrhoea are almost invariable in advanced uraemia. Restoration of menstruation following initiation of haemodialysis is common[147], though the menses are frequently irregular with metromenorrhagia and frequent anovulatory cycles[148,149]. Infertility is almost invariable in uraemic women while conception, when it does occur, is often followed by spontaneous abortion due to an inadequate luteal response to the pregnancy. Although pregnancy in uraemic women is rare it is usually undesirable for medical reasons, as there are major risks to the health of both mother and fetus if the pregnancy is allowed to proceed; the risk of spontaneous abortion with its associated morbidity and mortality is high. For these reasons it is desirable that all uraemic women in the childbearing age group be offered advice regarding contraception[150].

Sex hormones in uraemic women

Plasma levels of oestrogen and progesterone are usually low or low–normal in uraemic women while plasma LH and FSH are frequently raised[22,151]. Although LH and FSH are increased in premenopausal women with CRF, the increases are not parallel as in postmenopausal women, the most frequent pattern being a rise in LH and smaller rise in FSH[22]. This, of course, is the pattern of gonadotrophin excess seen in men with uraemia. Again the proposed explanation for these abnormalities is an alteration in set point for LH release. Uraemic women have normal gonadotrophin responses to LHRH and clomiphene suggesting that synthesis, storage and release of pituitary gonadotrophins are normal[22,152].

In healthy women gonadotrophins display cyclic changes with a surge of LH at ovulation (mid-cycle). This mid-cycle LH surge does not occur in uraemic women probably because positive oestradiol feedback on the hypothalamus is impaired. While failure of the LH surge undoubtedly contributes to menstrual problems in uraemic women, ovarian dysfunction is also of importance. In this context it has been observed that oestrogen levels fail to rise in mid-cycle or in response to clomiphene, even if there has been a naturally occurring or clomiphene-induced LH surge[22]. The mechanism of ovarian failure in uraemia remains obscure, though the observation that ovarian resistance to LH or HCG occurs in experimental uraemia suggests that direct inhibition of ovarian synthetic ability by unidentified 'uraemic toxins' may underlie the ovarian failure[153].

Hyperprolactinaemia

In patients with normal renal function, hyperprolactinaemia from a wide variety of causes has been associated with disordered sexual function, which is reversible by surgical or pharmacological control of the hyperprolactinaemia[154]. The mechanism whereby hyperprolactinaemia causes sexual dysfunction is disputed, being attributed either to central or peripheral effects on gonadotrophin release or function. In the context of uraemia the argument is largely academic: hyperprolactinaemia is common in uraemia, especially in women, and may therefore play an important role in the pathogenesis of sexual dysfunction in CRF[155–157]. Recognition of the contribution of hyperprolactinaemia to uraemic sexual problems is vital since treatment of the hyperprolactinaemia may improve symptoms of sexual dysfunction.

In addition to the symptoms outlined above, patients with hyperprolactinaemia may complain of galactorrhoea (in women)[158] or gynaecomastia (in men)[159]. The aetiology of uraemic hyperprolactinaemia involves both increased secretion and reduced degradation of prolactin[160]. Pituitary lactotrophs display resistance to suppression by dopamine or short-term administration of bromocriptine and impaired response to stimulation by TRH or chlorpromazine[155,156,161]. These abnormalities are suggestive of lactotroph autonomy which is not complete since plasma prolactin levels do fall appropriately in response to long-term therapy with bromocriptine, while administration of metoclopramide causes the expected increase in plasma prolactin[158,162,163].

Increased prolactin secretion in uraemia is often due to drugs such as methyldopa, metoclopramide or digoxin. Impaired metabolic clearance of prolactin does occur in uraemia but contributes little to hyperprolactinaemia; metabolic clearance is reported to be diminished by 33% in uraemic women with a four-fold increase in prolactin secretion rate[160].

Other factors

As suggested earlier, a wide range of non-hormonal mechanisms may contribute to disordered sexual dysfunction in CRF. Psychological factors such as anxiety, depression, stress or factors related specifically to CRF such as fear that sexual activity may in some way be harmful (e.g. to a CAPD catheter or kidney transplant) are frequently present and may either cause sexual dysfunction or aggravate a pre-existing organic problem[128,134]. Identification and, where possible, elimination of these problems is crucial in the management of sexual problems of uraemia.

Uraemic neuropathy or diabetic autonomic neuropathy are important to recognize as potential causes of impotence in men since the restoration of sexual function by renal transplant would be unlikely[128,164]. Similarly, vascular insufficiency is being increasingly recognized as a cause of irreversible impotence in uraemia[129]. Vascular insufficiency is most likely to occur in diabetics or in patients who have had both internal iliac arteries used for renal transplantation or who have atheroma affecting the pelvic vessels. In such patients penile blood flow is demonstrably impaired[129,165]. Attempts have been made at vascular reconstructive surgery as a therapy with some successes reported[165]. Many drugs, particularly anti-hypertensive agents, are also implicated as causes of reversible impotence in uraemia[133].

Zinc deficiency has been proposed as a treatable cause of sexual dysfunction in uraemia[130,131]. There is now reasonably good evidence that plasma or leukocyte zinc levels are low in CRF though the reason remains obscure. A recent report suggested that zinc absorption and retention was normal in uraemia while zinc elimination has not been reported to be enhanced[166]. It is possible that abnormalities noted in plasma zinc may represent altered distribution. Functionally, zinc is an important co-enzyme for a number of key enzymes including those involved in sex steroid biosynthesis[167]. There is therefore some physiological basis for the notion that zinc deficiency may cause sexual abnormalities by impairing sex steroid production. Unfortunately, the results of treating uraemic impotence with zinc are variable so that the association of zinc with sexual dysfunction remains unproven.

Diagnosis and management

The diagnosis and management of sexual dysfunction in uraemic men and women requires a clear understanding of the likely reversible cause. Drug induced, psychogenic and gonadal failure related causes are most likely to respond to therapy. It is equally important to identify those patients in whom a 'cure' is not likely since there may be alternative strategies that can be used in management.

The evaluation of a uraemic patient with sexual dysfunction should include a full history and physical examination, paying particular attention to evidence of neuropathy, vascular disease, psychogenic factors and details of sexual dysfunction. A full sexual history may be very difficult to obtain and may be facilitated by the use of a questionnaire. A drug history is clearly vital.

Serum concentrations of LH, FSH, prolactin and testosterone should be measured in the basal state in uraemic men. Sperm count and/or testicular biopsy may be important where the principal complaint is of infertility, particularly in predicting the response to therapy with FSH or renal transplant. In women LH, FSH, prolactin, oestradiol and progesterone should be measured during mid-cycle and again just prior to menstruation to assess luteal function.

If vascular insufficiency is suspected as a cause for impotence, penile blood flow can be measured by plethysmography or Doppler flow[168]. In selected cases, angiography with surgical or angioplastic reconstruction of arterial flow may improve impotence[165]. Where there is debate on the relative contributions of organic and psychogenic factors to impotence the evaluation of nocturnal penile tumescence (NPT) may be of assistance[169]. In true organic impotence nocturnal erections are reduced in both frequency and duration while in psychogenic impotence nocturnal erections are maintained. The frequent coincidence of both organic and psychogenic factors means that the routine use of NPT for evaluation of impotence in uraemia cannot be recommended.

Measurement of plasma zinc is of limited value in assessing uraemic gonadal dysfunction. Plasma zinc does not necessarily reflect tissue zinc[166], nor does it correlate consistently with either plasma testosterone or symptoms of hypogonadism. Leukocyte zinc correlates better both with plasma testosterone and with symptoms of hypogonadism but is not widely available. In practice it may be more reasonable to provide an oral zinc supplement for 6 months to patients suspected of being zinc deficient and to assess response in terms of both plasma testosterone and symptoms. There are few good controlled studies to support the routine use of zinc supplementation for hypogonadism[131] in uraemia but it seems reasonable to suggest its use in patients with low plasma testosterone levels and/or impotence. The suggested dose is zinc gluconate 25 mg daily by mouth. There is little evidence that zinc supplementation benefits sexual dysfunction in uraemic women.

Where hyperprolactinaemia is identified, a search should be made for a drug cause. Patients with drug-induced hyperprolactinaemia typically have extremely high serum prolactin concentrations and are more likely to have symptoms of prolactin excess. The offending drug(s) should be discontinued if possible[170]. Therapy with oral bromocriptine is successful in reducing serum prolactin to normal in the majority of patients, men and women, with uraemic hyperprolactinaemia[158,171]. Reduction in serum prolactin is associated with improvement in sexual dysfunction in both sexes. Bromocriptine therapy has been reported to improve impotence and lead to relatively normal concentrations of testosterone and gonadotrophin in men[171] and to improve menstrual irregularity and metromenorrhagia in uraemic women with hyperprolactinaemia[158].

CONCLUSION

The present chapter represents an attempt to encapsulate the often confusing array of endocrine abnormalities encountered in chronic renal failure and set them in the context of the uraemic syndrome. There is little doubt that some of these endocrine disorders contribute in a very major way to the symptoms of uraemia. Much remains to be learned, however, about the basis for disordered endocrine function in CRF and its clinical consequences.

References

1. Katz, A. I. and Rubenstein, A. H. (1973). Metabolism of proinsulin, insulin and C-peptide in the rat. *J. Clin. Invest.*, **52**, 1113–21
2. Emmanouel, D. S., Jaspan, J. B., Rubenstein, A. H. *et al.* (1978). Glucagon metabolism in the rat. Contribution of the kidney to the metabolic clearance rate of the hormone. *J. Clin. Invest.*, **62**, 6–13
3. Polonsky, K. S., Jaspan, J. B., Berlowitz, M. *et al.* (1981). Hepatic and renal metabolism of somatostatin-like immunoreactivity. Simultaneous assessment in the dog. *J. Clin. Invest.*, **68**, 1149–57
4. Hruska, K. A., Kopelman, R., Rutherford, E. *et al.* (1975). Metabolism of immunoreactive PTH in the dog. Role of the kidney and the effects of chronic renal disease. *J. Clin. Invest.*, **56**, 39–48
5. Ardaillou, R., Sizoneko, P., Meyrier, A. *et al.* (1970). Metabolic clearance rate of radioiodinated calcitonin in man. *J. Clin. Invest.*, **49**, 2345–52
6. Johnson, V. and Maack, T. (1977). Renal extraction, filtration, absorption and catabolism of growth hormone. *Am. J. Physiol.*, **233**, F173–8
7. Emmanouel, D. S., Fang, V. S. and Katz, A. I. (1981). Prolactin metabolism in the rat: role of the kidney in the degradation of the hormone. *Am. J. Physiol.*, **240**, F437–45
8. Arnaud, C. D. (1973). Hyperparathyroidism and renal failure. *Kidney Int.*, **4**, 89–95
9. Martin, K. J., Hruska, K. A., Freitag, J. J., Klahr, S. and Slatopolsky, E. (1979). The peripheral metabolism of parathyroid hormone. *N. Engl. J. Med.*, **301**, 1092–8
10. Adami, A., Muirhead, N., Manning, R. M. *et al.* (1982). Control of secretion of parathyroid hormone in secondary hyperparathyroidism. *Clin. Endocrinol.*, **16**, 463–73
11. Massry, S. G. (1979). Pathogenesis of secondary hyperparathyroidism in early renal failure: a multifactorial system including phosphate retention, skeletal resistance to PTH and altered vitamin D metabolism. In Norman, A. W. *et al.* (eds.), *Vitamin D, Basic Research and its Clinical Application. 4th International Workshop on Vitamin D*. p. 1203. (Berlin: De Gruyter)
12. Jaspan, J. B., Mako, M. E., Kuzuya, H. *et al.* (1977). Abnormalities in circulating beta cell peptides in chronic renal failure: comparison of C-peptide, proinsulin and insulin. *J. Clin. Endocrinol. Metab.*, **45**, 441–6
13. Rigopoulou, D., Valverde, I., Marco, J. *et al.* (1970). Large glucagon immunoreactivity in extracts of pancreas. *J. Biol. Chem.*, **245**, 496–501
14. Kuku, S. F., Jaspan, J. B., Emmanouel, D. S. *et al.* (1976). Heterogeneity of plasma glucagon. Circulating components in normal subjects and patients with chronic renal failure. *J. Clin. Invest.*, **58**, 742–50
15. Berl, T., Katz, F. H., Henrick, W. L. *et al.* (1978). Role of aldosterone in the

control of sodium excretion in patients with advanced chronic renal failure. *Kidney Int.*, **14,** 228–35
16. Hasegawa, K., Matsushita, Y., Inoue, T. *et al.* (1986). Plasma levels of atrial natriuretic peptide in patients with chronic renal failure. *J. Clin. Endocrinol. Metab.*, **63,** 819–22
17. Radtke, H.W., Erbes, P.M., Schippers, E. *et al.* (1978). Serum erythropoietin concentration in anephric patients. *Nephron,* **22,** 361–5
18. Caro, J., Brown, S., Miller, O., Murray, T. and Erslev, A.J. (1979). Erythropoietin levels in uremic nephric and anephric patients. *J. Lab. Clin. Med.*, **93,** 449–57
19. McGonigle, R.S., Wallin, J.D., Shadduck, R.K. and Fisher, J.W. (1984). Erythropoietin deficiency and inhibition of erythropoiesis in renal insufficiency. *Kidney Int.*, **25,** 437–44
20. Mason, R.S., Lissner, D., Wilkinson, M. and Posen, S. (1980). Vitamin D metabolites and their relationship to azotaemic osteodystrophy. *Clin. Endocrinol.*, **13,** 375–85
21. Chen, J.C., Vidt, D.G., Zorn, E.M. *et al.* (1970). Pituitary-Leydig cell function in uremic males. *J. Clin. Endocrinol.*, **31,** 14–17
22. Lim, V.S., Henriquez, C., Sievertsen, G. *et al.* (1980). Ovarian function in chronic renal failure: Evidence suggesting hypothalamic anovulation. *Ann. Intern. Med.*, **93,** 21–7
23. David, F.B., Spector, D.A., Davis, P.I. *et al.* (1982). Comparison of pituitary-thyroid function in patients with end-stage kidney disease and in age- and sex-matched controls. *Kidney Int.*, **21,** 362–4
24. Spector, D.A., Davis, P.J., Helderman, J.H. *et al.* (1976). Thyroid function and metabolic state in chronic renal failure. *Ann. Intern. Med.*, **85,** 724–30
25. Lim, V.S., Fang, V.S., Katz, A.I. *et al.* (1977). Thyroid dysfunction in chronic renal failure. A study of the pituitary-thyroid axis and peripheral turnover kinetics of thyroxine and triiodothyronine. *J. Clin. Invest.*, **60,** 522–34
26. Massry, S.G., Stein, R., Garty, J. *et al.* (1976). Skeletal resistance to the calcemic action of PTH in ureamia – a role of 1,25 dihydroxycholecalciferol. *Kidney Int.*, **9,** 467–74
27. Smith, S., Anderson, S., Ballerman, B.J. *et al.* (1986). Role of atrial natriuretic peptide in adaptation of sodium excretion to reduced nephron mass. *J. Clin. Invest.*, **77,** 1395–8
28. De Fronzo, R.A., Alvestrand, A., Smith, D. *et al.* (1981). Insulin resistance in uraemia. *J. Clin. Invest.*, **67,** 563–8
29. Dandona, P., Newton, D. and Platts, M.M. (1977). Long-term hemodialysis and renal function. *Br. Med. J.*, **1,** 134–6
30. Silverberg, D.S., Ulan, R.A., Fawcett, D.M. *et al.* (1973). Effect of chronic hemodialysis on thyroid function in chronic renal failure. *Can. Med. Assoc. J.*, **109,** 282–6
31. Chopra, I.J., Chopra, U., Smith, S.R. *et al.* (1975). Reciprocal changes in serum concentration of 3,3′,5-triiodothyronine (reverse T_3) and 3,3′,5-triiodothyronine (T_3) in systemic illness. *J. Clin. Endocrinol. Metab.*, **41,** 1043–9
32. Utiger, R.D. (1980). Decreased extrathyroidal triiodothyronine production in non-thyroidal illness: benefit or harm? *Am. J. Med.*, **69,** 807–10
33. Carter, J.N., Eastman, C.J., Corcoran, J.M. *et al.* (1977). Effect of triiodothyronine administration in patients with chronic renal failure. *Aust. N.Z.J. Med.*, **7,** 612–16

34. Melmed, S., Geola, F. L., Reed, A. W. *et al.* (1982). A comparison of methods for assessing thyroid function in non-thyroidal illness. *J. Clin. Endocrinol. Metab.*, **54**, 300–6
35. Blair, A. J., Morgan, R. O. and Beck, J. C. (1961). The plasma 17-hydroxy-corticosteroid levels in acute and chronic renal failure. *Can. J. Biochem.*, **39**, 1617–24
36. Englert, E., Brown, H., Williamson, D. G. *et al.* (1958). Metabolism of free and conjugated 17-hydroxycorticosteroids in subjects with uraemia. *J. Clin. Endocrinol. Metab.*, **18**, 36–48
37. Wallace, E. Z., Rosman, P., Toshav, N. *et al.* (1980). Pituitary-adrenocortical function in chronic renal failure: studies of episodic secretion of cortisol and dexamethasone suppressibility. *J. Clin. Endocrinol. Metab.*, **50**, 46–51
38. Mishkin, M. S., Hsu, T. H., Walker, W. G. *et al.* (1972). Studies on the episodic secretion of cortisone in uraemic patients on hemodialysis. *Johns Hopkins Med. J.*, **131**, 161–4
39. Tsuchida, S., Sugawara, H. and Fukuchi, S. (1970). Plasma cortisol level during hemodialysis with Kolff's artificial kidney. *Tohoku J. Exp. Med.*, **100**, 23–9
40. Akmal, M. and Manzler, A. D. (1977). Simplified assessment of pituitary-adrenal axis in a stable group of chronic hemodialysis patients. *Trans. Am. Soc. Artif. Intern. Organs*, **23**, 730–6
41. Feldman, H. A. and Singer, I. (1974). Endocrinology and metabolism in uremia and dialysis: a clinical review. *Medicine*, **54**, 345–76
42. Rosman, P. M., Farag, A. and Peckham, R. (1982). Pituitary-adrenocortical function in chronic renal failure: blunted suppression and early escape of plasma cortisol levels after intravenous dexamethasone. *J. Clin. Endocrinol. Metab.*, **54**, 528–33
43. McDonald, W. J., Golper, T. A., Mass, R. D. *et al.* (1979). Adrenocorticotrophin–cortisol axis abnormalities in hemodialysis patients. *J. Clin. Endocrinol. Metab.*, **48**, 92–5
44. Aronin, N., Liotta, A. S., Shickmanter, B. *et al.* (1981). Impaired clearance of β-lipotrophin in uremia. *J. Clin. Endocrinol. Metab.*, **53**, 797–800
45. Krieger, D. T., Liotta, A. S., Suda, T. *et al.* (1979). Human plasma immunoreactive lipotropin and adrenocorticotropin in normal subjects and in patients with pituitary-adrenal disease. *J. Clin. Endocrinol. Metab.*, **48**, 566–71
46. Ramirez, G., Etheridge, W., Meikle, W. *et al.* (1978). Evaluation of the pituitary adrenal axis in patients with chronic renal failure. *Clin. Res.*, **26**, 148
47. Smith, A. G., Shuster, S., Comaish, J. S. *et al.* (1975). Plasma immunoreactive melanocyte-stimulating hormone and skin pigmentation in chronic renal failure. *Br. Med. J.*, **1**, 658–9
48. Gold, E. M., Kleeman, C. R., Ling, S., Yawata, M. N. and Maxwell, M. (1965). Sustained aldosterone secretion in chronic renal failure. *Clin. Res.*, **13**, 135A
49. Oh, M. S., Carroll, H. J., Clemmons, J. E., Vagnucci, A. H., Levinson, S. P. and Whang, E. S. N. (1974). A mechanism for hyporeninemic hypoaldosteronism in chronic renal disease. *Metabolism*, **23**, 1157–66
50. De Fronzo, R. (1980). Hyperkalemia and hyporeninemic hypoaldosteronism. *Kidney Int.*, **17**, 118–34
51. Bricker, N. S. (1967). The control of sodium excretion with normal and reduced nephron populations: the pre-eminence of third factor. *Am. J. Med.*, **43**, 313–21

52. Cole, B. R., Kuhnline, M. A. and Needleman, P. (1985). Atriopeptin III. A potent natriuretic, diuretic and hypotensive agent in rats with chronic renal failure. *J. Clin. Invest.*, **76,** 2413–15
53. Kahn, T., Kaji, D. M., Nicolis, G., Krakoff, L. R. and Stein, R. M. (1978). Factors related to potassium transport in stable chronic renal disease. *Clin. Sci. Mol. Med.*, **54,** 661–6
54. McGonigle, R. S., Wallin, J. D., Shadduck, R. K. and Fisher, J. W. (1984). Erythropoietin deficiency and inhibition of erythropoiesis in renal insufficiency. *Kidney Int.*, **25,** 437–44
55. Erslev, A. J., Caro, J., Miller, O. and Silver, R. (1980). Plasma erythropoietin in health and disease. *Ann. Lab. Clin. Sci.*, **10,** 250–7
56. Eschbach, J. W., Egrie, J. C., Downing, M. R. *et al.* (1987). Correction of the anemia of end-stage renal disease with recombinant human erythropoietin. Results of a combined phase I and phase II clinical trial. *N. Engl. J. Med.*, **316,** 713–18
57. Winearls, C. G., Oliver, D. O., Pippard, M. J., Reid, C., Downing, M. R. and Cotes, P. M. (1986). Effect of human erythropoietin derived from recombinant DNA on the anemia of patients maintained by chronic hemodialysis. *Lancet*, **2,** 1175–8
58. Eschbach, J. W. and Adamson, J. W. (1973). Improvement in the anemia of chronic renal failure with fluoxymesterone. *Ann. Intern. Med.*, **78,** 527–30
59. Linton, A. L., Clark, W. F., Dreidger, A. A., Werb, R. and Lindsay, R. M. (1977). Correctable factors contributing to the anemia of dialysis patients. *Nephron*, **19,** 95–8
60. Muirhead, N., Keown, P. A. K., Hollomby, D. J. *et al.* (1988). A randomised, double-blind trial of r-HuEPO in the anemia of chronic renal failure. (Manuscript in preparation)
61. Reiss, E. and Canterbury, J. M. (1971). Genesis of hyperparathyroidism. *Am. J. Med.*, **50,** 679–85
62. Slatopolsky, E. and Bricker, N. S. (1973). The role of phosphorus restriction in the prevention of secondary hyperparathyroidism in chronic renal disease. *Kidney Int.*, **4,** 141–5
63. Malluche, H. H., Ritz, E., Lange, H. P. *et al.* (1975). Bone histology in incipient and advanced renal failure. *Kidney Int.*, **9,** 355–62
64. Massry, S. G. and Ritz, E. (1978). The pathogenesis of secondary hyperparathyroidism of renal failure. Is there a controversy? *Arch. Intern. Med.*, **138,** 853–6
65. Slatopolsky, E., Gray, R., Adams, N. D. *et al.* (1979). Pathogenesis of secondary hyperparathyroidism in early chronic renal failure. In Norman, A. W. *et al.* (eds.), *Vitamin D, Basic Research and Its Clinical Application. 4th International Workshop on Vitamin D.* p. 1209. (Berlin: DeGruyter)
66. Freitag, J., Martin, K. J., Hruska, K. *et al.* (1978). Impaired parathyroid hormone metabolism in patients with chronic renal failure. *N. Engl. J. Med.*, **298,** 29–32
67. Berlyne, G. M., Ben-Arie, J., Epstein, N., Booth, E..M. and Yagil, R. (1973). Rarity of renal osteodystrophy in Israel is due to low phosphorus intake. *Nephron*, **10,** 141–56
68. Bouillon, R., Verberckmoes, R. and De Moor, P. (1975). Influence of dialysate

calcium concentration and vitamin D on parathyroid hormone during repetitive dialysis. *Kidney Int.*, **7**, 422–32
69. Ritz, E., Malluche, H. H., Krempien, B. and Mehls, O. (1977). Bone histology in renal failure In David, D. S. (ed.), *Calcium Metabolism in Renal Failure and Nephrolithiasis*. p. 197. (New York: Wiley)
70. Coburn, J. W., Brickman, A. S., Sherrard, D. *et al.* (1977). Use of 1,25$(OH)_2$ vitamin D_3 to separate 'types' of renal osteodystrophy. *Proc. Eur. Dial. Transplant Assoc.*, **14**, 442–50
71. Slatopolsky, E., Rutherford, W. E., Hoffstein, P. E. *et al.* (1972). Non-suppressible secondary hyperparathyroidism in chronic progressive renal disease. *Kidney Int.*, **1**, 38–46
72. David, D. S., Sakai, S., Brennan, B. L. *et al.* (1973). Hypercalcemia after renal transplantation. *N. Engl. J. Med.*, **289**, 398–401
73. Christensen, M. S. and Nielson, H. E. (1977). Parathyroid function after renal transplantation. Interrelationships between renal function, serum calcium and serum parathyroid hormone in normocalcemic long-term survivors. *Clin. Nephrol.*, **8**, 472–6
74. Goldstein, D. A., Malluche, H. H. and Massry, S. G. (1979). Management of renal osteodystrophy with 1,25$(OH)_2$ vitamin D_3. *Min. Elect. Metab.*, **2**, 35–47
75. Massry, S. G. and Goldstein, D. A. (1979). The search for uremic toxin(s) 'X'. 'X' = PTH. *Clin. Nephrol.*, **11**, 181–9
76. Massry, S. G. (1985). Neurotoxicity of parathyroid hormone in uremia. *Kidney Int.*, **28**, (S17), 505–11
77. Wallach, S., Ballavia, J. V., Shorr, J. and Schaffers, J. (1966). Tissue distributions of electrolyte, Ca^{47} and Mg^{28} in experimental hyper- and hypoparathyroidism. *Endocrinology*, **78**, 16–28
78. Goldstein, D. A. and Massry, S. G. (1978). Effect of parathyroid hormone administration and its withdrawal on brain calcium and electroencephalogram. *Min. Elect. Metab.*, **1**, 84–92
79. Fioretti, P., Melis, G. B., Ciardella, F. *et al.* (1986). Parathyroid function and pituitary-gonadal axis in male uremic: effects of dietary treatment and of maintenance hemodialysis. *Clin. Nephrol.*, **25**, 155–8
80. Drueke, T., Fauchet, M., Fleury, J. *et al.* (1980). Effect of parathyroidectomy on left ventricular function in haemodialysis patients. *Lancet*, **1**, 112–14
81. Collins, J., Massry, S. G. and Campese, V. M. (1985). Parathyroid hormone and the altered vascular response to norepinephrine in uraemia. *Am. J. Nephrol.*, **5**, 110–13
82. Saglikes, Y., Massry, S. G., Iseki, K., Nadler, J. L. and Campese, V. M. (1985). Effect of PTH on blood pressure and response to vasoconstrictor agonists. *Am. J. Physiol.*, **248**, F674–81
83. Bogin, E., Massry, S. G., Levi, J., Djaldeti, M., Bristol, G. and Smith, J. (1982). Effects of parathyroid hormone on osmotic fragility of human erythrocytes. *J. Clin. Invest.*, **69**, 1017–25
84. Saltissi, D. and Carter, G. D. (1985). Association of secondary hyperparathyroidism with red cell survival in chronic hemodialysis patients. *Clin. Sci.*, **18**, 29–33
85. Weinberg, S. G., Lubin, A., Weiner, S. N. *et al.* (1977). Myelofibrosis and renal osteodystrophy. *Am. J. Med.*, **63**, 755–64
86. Lutton, J. D., Solangi, K. B., Ibrahim, N. G., Goodman, A. I. and Levere,

R. D. (1984). Inhibition of erythropoietin in chronic renal failure: the role of parathyroid hormone. *Am. J. Kid. Dis.*, **3,** 380–4
87. Remuzzi, G., Dodesini, P., Livio, M. *et al.* (1981). Parathyroid hormone inhibits human platelet function.. *Lancet,* **2,** 1321–3
88. Docci, D., Turci, F., Delvecchio, C., Gollini, G., Baldrati, L. and Pistocchi, E. (1986). Lack of evidence for the role of secondary hyperparathyroidism in the pathogenesis of uremic thrombocytopathy. *Nephron,* **43,** 28–32
89. DeBold, A. J. (1985). Atrial natriuretic factor: a hormone produced by the heart. *Science,* **230,** 767–70
90. Ballerman, B. J. and Brenner, B. M. (1985). Biologically active atrial peptides. *J. Clin. Invest.*, **76,** 2041–8
91. Ballerman, B. J. and Brenner, B. M. (1986). Role of atrial peptides in body fluid homeostasis. *Circ. Res.*, **58,** 620–30
92. Maack, T., Marion, D. N., Camargo, M. J. *et al.* (1984). Effects of auriculin (atrial natriuretic factor) on blood pressure, renal function and the renin-angiotensin system in dogs. *Am. J. Med.*, **77,** 1069–77
93. Zeidel, M. L. and Brenner, B. (1987). Actions of atrial natriuretic peptides on the kidney. *Sem. Nephrol.*, **7,** 91–7
94. Sonnenberg, H., Cupples, W. A., DeBold, A. J. *et al.* (1982). Intrarenal localization of the natriuretic effect of cardiac atrial extract. *Can. J. Physiol. Pharmacol.*, **60,** 1149–52
95. Horton, E. S., Johnson, C. and Lebovitz, H. E. (1968). Carbohydrate metabolism in uremia. *Ann. Intern. Med.*, **68,** 63–74
96. DeFronzo, R. A., Andres, R., Edgar, P. *et al.* (1973). Carbohydrate metabolism in uremia: a review. *Medicine,* **52,** 469–81
97. Cerletty, J. M. and Engbring, N. H. (1967). Azotemia and glucose intolerance. *Ann. Intern. Med.*, **66,** 1097–108
98. Bagdade, J. D., Porte, D. and Bierman, E. L. (1968). Hypertriglyceridemia. A metabolic consequence of chronic renal failure. *N. Engl. J. Med.*, **279,** 181–5
99. Lowrie, E. G., Soeldner, J. S., Hampers, C. L. *et al.* (1970). Glucose metabolism and insulin secretion in uremic, prediabetic and normal subjects. *J. Lab. Clin. Med.*, **76,** 603–15
100. Spitz, I. M., Rubenstein, A. H., Bersohn, I. *et al.* (1970). Carbohydrate metabolism in renal disease. *Q. J. Med.*, **89,** 201–26
101. Navalesi, R., Pilo, A., Lenzi, S. *et al.* (1975). Insulin metabolism in chronic uremia and in the anephric state: effect of the dialytic treatment. *J. Clin. Endocrinol. Metab.*, **40,** 70–85
102. Mondon, C. E., Dolkas, C. B. and Reaven, G. M. (1978). Effect of acute uremia on insulin removal by the isolated perfused rat liver and muscle. *Metabolism,* **27,** 133–42
103. Runyan, R. W., Hurwitz, D. and Robbins, S. L. (1955). Effect of Kimmelstiel–Wilson syndrome on insulin requirements in diabetes. *N. Engl. J. Med.*, **252,** 385–91
104. Zubrod, C. G., Eversole, S. L. and Dana, G. W. (1951). Amelioration of diabetes and striking rarity of acidosis in patients with Kimmelstiel–Wilson lesions. *N. Engl. J. Med.*, **245,** 518–25
105. Frizzel, M., Larsen, P. R. and Field, J. B. (1973). Spontaneous hypoglycemia associated with chronic renal failure. *Diabetes,* **22,** 493–8
106. Garber, A. J. and Bier, D. M., Cryer, P. E. *et al.* (1974). Hypoglycemia in

compensated chronic renal failure. Substrate limitation of gluconeogenesis. *Diabetes*, **23,** 982–6
107. Owen, O. E., Felig, P., Morgan, A. P., Wahren, J. and Cahill, G. F. (1969). Liver and kidney metabolism during prolonged starvation. *J. Clin. Invest.*, **48,** 574–83
108. Pun, K. K., Yeung, C. K., Ho, P. W. M., Lin, H. J., Chan, J. K. and Yeung, M. T. T. (1984). Effects of propranolol and haemodialysis on the response of glucose, insulin, C-peptide and cyclic AMP to glucagon challenge. *Clin. Nephrol.*, **21,** 235–40
109. DeFronzo, R. A., Alvestrand, A., Smith, D. *et al.* (1981). Insulin resistance in uremia. *J. Clin. Invest.*, **67,** 563–81
110. Westervelt, F. B. (1969). Insulin effect in uremia. *J. Lab. Clin. Med.*, **74,** 79–84
111. Smith, D. and DeFronzo, R. A. (1982). Insulin resistance in uremia mediated by post-binding defects. *Kidney Int.*, **22,** 54–62
112. Hampers, C. L., Soeldner, J. S., Doak, P. B. *et al.* (1966). Effect of chronic renal failure and hemodialysis on carbohydrate metabolism. *J. Clin. Invest.*, **45,** 1719–31
113. Alfrey, A. C., Sussman, K. E. and Holmes, J. H. (1967). Changes in glucose and insulin metabolism induced by dialysis in patients with chronic uremia. *Metabolism*, **16,** 733–40
114. Orskov, H. and Christensen, N. J. (1971). Growth hormone in uremia. I. Plasma growth hormone, insulin and glucagon after oral and intravenous glucose in uremic subjects. *Scand. J. Clin. Lab. Invest.*, **27,** 51–60
115. Samaan, N. and Freeman, R. M. (1970). Growth hormone levels in severe renal failure. *Metabolism*, **19,** 102–13
116. Bilbrey, G. L., Faloona, G. R., White, M. G. *et al.* (1974). Hyperglucagonemia of renal failure. *J. Clin. Invest.*, **53,** 841–7
117. Kuku, S. F., Jaspan, J. B., Emmanouel, D. S. *et al.* (1976). Heterogeneity of plasma glucagon. Circulating components in normal subjects and patients with chronic renal failure. *J. Clin. Invest.*, **58,** 742–50
118. Kuku, S. F., Zeidler, A., Emmanouel, D. S. *et al.* (1976). Heterogeneity of plasma glucagon: patterns in patients with chronic renal failure and diabetes. *J. Clin. Endocrinol. Metab.*, **42,** 173–6
119. Brunzell, J. D., Albers, J. J., Hass, L. B. *et al.* (1977). Prevalence of serum lipid abnormalities in chronic hemodialysis. *Metabolism*, **26,** 903–10
120. Ibels, L. S., Simons, L. A., King, J. O. *et al.* (1975). Studies on the nature and causes of hyperlipidemia in uremia, maintenance dialysis and renal transplantation. *Q. J. Med.*, **24,** 501–14
121. Cattran, D. C., Fenton, S. S. A., Wilson, D. R. *et al.* (1976). Defective triglyceride removal in lipemia associated with peritoneal dialysis and hemodialysis. *Ann. Intern. Med.*, **85,** 29–33
122. Nicholls, A. J., Catto, G. R. D., Edward, N., Engeset, J. and MacLeod, M. (1980). Accelerated atherosclerosis in long-term dialysis and renal transplant patients: fact or fiction? *Lancet*, **1,** 276–8
123. Shepherd, A. M. M., Stewart, W. K. and Wormsley, K. G. (1973). Peptic ulceration in chronic renal disease. *Lancet*, **1,** 1957–9
124. Korman, M. G., Laver, M. C. and Hansky, L. (1972). Hypergastrinemia in chronic renal failure. *Br. Med. J.*, **1,** 209–10
125. Muto, S., Murayama, N., Asano, Y., Hosoda, S. and Miyata, M. (1985).

Hypergastrinemia and achlorhydria in chronic renal failure. *Nephron,* **40,** 143–8
126. El Ghounaimy, E., Barsoum, R., Soliman, M. *et al.* (1985). Serum gastrin in chronic renal failure: morphological and physiological considerations. *Nephron,* **39,** 86–94
127. Andriulli, A., Malfi, B., Recchia, S., Ponti, V., Triolo, G. and Segoloni, G. (1985). Patients with chronic renal failure are not at a risk of developing chronic peptic ulcers. *Clin. Nephrol.,* **23,** 245–8
128. Levy, N. B. and Wynbrandt, G. D. (1975). The quality of life on maintenance hemodialysis. *Lancet,* **1,** 1328–30
129. Degen, K., Strain, J. J. and Zurnoff, B. (1983). Biopsychosocial evaluation of sexual function in end-stage renal disease. In *Psychonephrology.* p. 23. (New York: Plenum)
130. Antoniou, L. D., Shalhoub, R. J., Sudhakar, T. and Smith, J. C. (1977). Reversal of uraemic impotence by zinc. *Lancet,* **2,** 895–8
131. Mahajan, S., Abbasi, A. A., Prasad, A. S. *et al.* (1982). Effect of oral zinc therapy on gonadal function in hemodialysis patients. A double blind study. *Ann. Intern. Med.,* **97,** 357–61
132. Thurm, J. (1975). Sexual potency in patients on hemodialysis. *Urology,* **5,** 60–4
133. Procci, W. R., Goldstein, D. A., Kletzky, O. A., Campese, V. M. and Massry, S. G. (1983). Impotence in uremia. In Levy, N. B. (ed.), *Psychonephrology.* p. 235 (New York: Plenum)
134. Levy, N. B. (1973). Sexual adjustment of maintenance hemodialysis and renal transplantation: national survey by questionnaire: preliminary report. *Trans. Am. Soc. Artif. Intern. Organs,* **19,** 138–43
135. Bailey, G. L. (1977). The sick kidney and sex. *N. Engl. J. Med.,* **296,** 1288–9
136. Larsen, N. R. (1972). Sexual problems of patients on RDT and after renal transplantation. *Proc. Eur. Dial. Transpl. Assoc.,* **9,** 271–7
137. Mastrogiacomo, I., De Besi, L., Serafini, E. *et al.* (1984). Hyperprolactinemia and menstrual disturbances among uremic women on hemodialysis. *Nephron,* **37,** 195–9
138. Lim, V. S. and Fang, V. S. (1975). Gonadal dysfunction in uremic men. A study of the hypothalamo-pituitary-testicular axis before and after renal transplantation. *Am. J. Med.,* **58,** 655–62
139. De Kretsker, D. M., Atkins, R. C. and Scott, D. F. (1974). Disordered spermatogenesis in patients with chronic renal failure undergoing maintenance hemodialysis. *Aust. N.Z. J. Med.,* **4,** 178–81
140. Rager, K., Bundschu, H. and Gupta, D. (1975). The effect of HCG on testicular androgen production in adult men with chronic renal failure. *J. Reprod. Fertil.,* **42,** 113–20
141. Stewart-Bentley, M., Gans, D. and Horton, R. (1974). Regulation of gonadal function in uremia. *Metabolism,* **23,** 1065–72
142. Holdsworth, S. R., DeKretser, D. M. and Atkins, R. C. (1978). A comparison of hemodialysis and transplantation in reversing the uremic disturbances of male reproductive function. *Clin. Nephrol.,* **10,** 146–50
143. Zumoff, B., Walter, L., Rosenfeld, R. S. *et al.* (1980). Subnormal plasma adrenal androgen levels in men with uremia. *J. Clin. Endocrinol. Metab.,* **51,** 801–5
144. Holdsworth, S., Atkins, R. C. and DeKretsker, D. M. (1977). The pituitary-testicular axis in men with chronic renal failure. *N. Engl. J. Med.,* **296,** 1245–9

145. Guevara, A., Vidt, A., Fallberg, M. C. *et al.* (1969). Serum gonadotrophins and testosterone levels in uremic males undergoing intermittent dialysis. *Metabolism*, **18**, 1062–6
146. Lim, V. S. and Fang, V. S. (1976). Restoration of plasma testosterone levels in uremic men with clomiphene citrate. *J. Clin. Endocrinol. Metab.*, **43**, 1370–7
147. Merkatz, I. R., Schwartz, G. H., David, S. *et al.* (1971). Resumption of female reproductive function following renal transplantation. *J. Am. Med. Assoc.*, **216**, 1749–54
148. Wass, V. I., Wass, J. A. H., Rees, L. *et al.* (1978). Sex hormone changes underlying menstrual disturbances on hemodialysis. *Proc. Eur. Dial. Transpl. Assoc.*, **15**, 178–86
149. Zingraff, J., Jungers, P., Pelissier, C. *et al.* (1982). Pituitary and ovarian dysfunction in women on hemodialysis. *Nephron*, **30**, 149–53
150. Goodwin, N. J., Valenti, C., Hall, J. E. *et al.* (1968). Effects of uremia and chronic hemodialysis on the reproductive cycle. *Am. J. Obstet. Gynecol.*, **100**, 528–35
151. Strickler, R. C., Woolever, C. A., Johnson, M. *et al.* (1974). Serum gonadotrophin patterns in patients with chronic renal failure on hemodialysis. *Gynecol. Invest.*, **5**, 185–98
152. Swamy, A. P., Woolf, P. D. and Cestero, R. F. (1979). Hypothalamic-pituitary-ovarian axis in uremic women. *J. Lab. Clin. Med.*, **93**, 1066–72
153. Kreusser, W., Mader, H., Waag, W. D. *et al.* (1982). Diminished response of ovarian cAMP to luteinizing hormone in experimental uremia. *Kidney Int.*, **22**, 272–9
154. Spark, R. F. and Dickstein, G. (1979). Bromocriptine and endocrine disorders. *Ann. Intern. Med.*, **90**, 949–56
155. Ramirez, G., O'Neill, W. M., Bloomer, H. A. *et al.* (1977). Abnormalities in the regulation of prolactin in patients with chronic renal failure. *J. Clin. Endocrinol. Metab.*, **45**, 658–61
156. Lim, V. S., Kathpalia, S. C. and Frohman, L. A. (1979). Hyperprolactinemia and impaired pituitary response to suppression and stimulation in chronic renal failure: reversal after transplantation. *J. Clin. Endocrinol. Metab.*, **48**, 101–7
157. Cowden, E. A., Ratcliffe, W. A., Ratcliffe, J. G. *et al.* (1978). Hyperprolactinemia in renal disease. *Clin. Endocrinol.*, **9**, 241–8
158. Gomez, F., De La Cueva, R., Wauters, J. P. *et al.* (1980). Endocrine abnormalities in patients undergoing long-term hemodialysis. The role of prolactin. *Am. J. Med.*, **68**, 522–30
159. Freeman, P. M., Lawton, R. L. and Fearing, M. O. (1968). Gynaecomastia: an endocrinologic complication of hemodialysis. *Ann. Intern. Med.*, **69**, 67–72
160. Sieversten, G. D., Lim, V. S., Nakawatese, C. *et al.* (1980). Metabolic clearance and secretion rates of human prolactin in normal subjects and in patients with chronic renal failure. *J. Clin. Endocrinol. Metab.*, **50**, 846–52
161. Peces, R., Horcajada, C., Lopez-Noroa, M. J. *et al.* (1981). Hyperprolactinemia in chronic renal failure: impaired responsiveness to stimulation and suppression. *Nephron*, **28**, 11–16
162. Bommer, J., Del Pozo, E., Ritz, E. *et al.* (1979). Improved sexual function in male hemodialysis patients on bromocriptine. *Lancet*, **2**, 496–7
163. Leroith, D., Danovitz, G., Trestan, S. *et al.* (1979). Dissociation of prolactin

response to thyrotropin-releasing hormone and metoclopramide in chronic renal failure. *J. Clin. Endocrinol. Metab.*, **49,** 815–17
164. Bommer, J., Tschoppe, W., Ritz, E. *et al.* (1976). Sexual behaviour of hemodialysis patients. *Clin. Nephrol.*, **6,** 315–18
165. Hawatmeh, I. S., Houttuin, E., Gregory, J. G., Blair, O. M. and Purcell, M. H. (1982). The diagnosis and surgical management of vasculogenic impotence. *J. Urol.*, **127,** 910–14
166. Muirhead, N., Kertesz, A., Flanagan, P. R., Hodsman, A. B., Hollomby, D. J. and Valberg, L. S. (1986). Zinc metabolism in patients on maintenance hemodialysis. *Am. J. Nephrol.*, **6,** 422–6
167. Ulmer, D. D. (1977). Trace elements. *N. Engl. J. Med.*, **297,** 318–21
168. Michal, V. and Popischal, J. (1978). Phalloarteriography in the diagnosis of erectile impotence. *World J. Surg.*, **2,** 239–48
169. Marshall, P., Surridge, D. and Delva, N. (1981). The role of nocturnal penile tumescence in differentiating between organic and psychogenic impotence; the first stage of validation. *Arch. Sex. Behav.*, **10,** 1–10
170. Hou, S. H., Grossman, S. and Molitch, M. E. (1985). Hyperprolactinemia in patients with renal insufficiency and chronic renal failure requiring hemodialysis or chronic ambulatory peritoneal dialysis. *Am. J. Kid. Dis.*, **4,** 245–9
171. Ermolenko, V. M., Kukhtevitch, A. K., Dedov, I. I., Bunation, A. F., Melnichenko, G. A. and Gitel, E. P. (1986). Parlodel treatment of uremic hypogonadism in men. *Nephron,* **42,** 19–22

4

BONE DISEASE IN CHRONIC RENAL FAILURE

A. J. FELSENFELD AND F. LLACH

Altered bone pathology has been observed in patients with chronic renal failure since the early 1900s[1]. The association between chronic renal failure and the development of bone disease was established during the first half of this century[2,3]. During the 1930s, parathyroid hyperplasia was described in patients with renal failure[4–6]. Subsequently, with the advent of the radioimmunoassay in the 1960s, elevated parathyroid hormone (PTH) levels were documented in renal failure[7–9]. However, in general, overt skeletal disease did not become a serious clinical problem until the widespread availability of maintenance dialysis during the last two decades. It became apparent that dialytic therapy did not correct the skeletal disease; neither did the reduction of excess PTH, as a result of parathyroidectomy. Furthermore, the correction of the vitamin D deficiency with the active metabolite, 1,25 dihydroxyvitamin D_3 (1,25$(OH)_2$D) also failed to restore bone histology to normal. Both of these treatment modalities have appropriate applications, but renal osteodystrophy has proved to be more complicated than an excess and deficiency state. From the perspective of today's clinician, the existence of several types of renal bone disease must be appreciated and treatment adapted to the type of bone disease and the individual needs of the patient.

FACTORS CONTRIBUTING TO THE DEVELOPMENT OF SECONDARY HYPERPARATHYROIDISM

Secondary hyperparathyroidism is the single factor most responsible for changes in bone histology in renal failure. Increased circulating levels of PTH and the presence of hyperplasia of the parathyroid gland have been observed in early and advanced renal failure[4–9]. The precise reason or reasons for these findings remain a subject of investigation.

Until recently, the consensus of opinion was that the presence of hypocalcaemia was the primary stimulus for the development of hyperparathyroidism. Several hypotheses were advanced as to the cause of the hypocalcaemia. The concept that phosphate retention was a primary cause of hyperparathyroidism was developed in the late 1960s and early 1970s[9–11]. This hypothesis, known as the trade-off hypothesis, held that in early renal failure a mild increase in serum phosphate develops because of decreased phosphate excretion secondary to the decline in the glomerular filtration rate. As the serum phosphate increases, hypocalcaemia ensues leading to an increase in PTH secretion. The increased PTH levels, because of PTH's phosphaturic effect and ability to reclaim skeletal calcium, re-establish normal serum calcium and phosphate levels. However, this normalization of serum calcium and phosphate is achieved at the cost of higher basal PTH levels. Thus, the term trade-off hypothesis is derived. With continued decline in glomerular filtration rate, a repetition of the above events occurs until the glomerular filtration rate declines to approximately 20–25 ml/min; then overt hyperphosphataemia develops despite marked elevation of PTH[12].

The trade-off hypothesis was derived from experimental data which showed that phosphate restriction prevented the development of hyperparathyroidism in the dog with surgically induced, advanced renal failure[10]. Recently it has been observed that phosphate restriction increases serum $1,25(OH)_2D$ production[13,14], which in turn may directly inhibit PTH secretion[15–17] (see later discussion) and increase calcium absorption from the gut[18,19]. The development of hyperparathyroidism in early renal failure may be due to factors other than phosphate retention. In fact, hypophosphataemia rather than hyperphosphataemia has been the predominant finding[20–22]. Even the hypothesis of post-prandial hyperphosphataemia when assessed by phosphate loading has not been verified, rather increased phosphaturia without hyperphosphataemia has been observed[22,23]. Finally, a recent *in vitro* study has shown that mild hyperphosphataemia does not produce hypocalcaemia[24].

In advanced renal failure, overt hyperphosphataemia probably plays an important role in the hyperparathyroidism[25,26]. Furthermore, a study in animals has suggested that the hyperphosphataemia can directly inhibit calcium release from bone[27]. This could theoretically exacerbate the hyperparathyroidism.

An abnormal vitamin D metabolism may play an important role in the pathogenesis of secondary hyperparathyroidism. Vitamin D is formed endogenously in the skin when 7-dehydrocholesterol is activated by ultraviolet light. The vitamin D, synthesized in the skin and derived from dietary sources, is transported to the liver where 25-hydroxylation occurs. This process of 25-hydroxylation is poorly regulated and thus is a good index of vitamin D reserves[28]. The hormonal form of vitamin D, $1,25(OH)_2D$, is formed in the mitochondria of the proximal tubules of the kidney where 25(OH)D undergoes 1α-hydroxylation[29]. Major factors regulating the enzymatic conversion to $1,25(OH)_2D$ include PTH[30,31] as well as the concentration of serum phosphate[32,33] and serum calcium[34,35]. Thus, high levels of PTH, hypophosphataemia, and hypocalcaemia stimulate the production of $1,25(OH)_2D$. The concentration of $1,25(OH)_2D$ is low in advanced renal failure[36,37]. In early renal failure, both decreased[22,23] and normal [14,38] levels of $1,25(OH)_2D$ have been reported and these levels are stimulated by phosphate restriction[13,14].

The progressively lower levels of $1,25(OH)_2D$ observed in renal failure affect mineral and skeletal metabolism. Thus, $1,25(OH)_2D$ may have a direct effect on both the action and secretion of PTH. Such examples include an improved calcaemic response of PTH after $1,25(OH)_2D$ administration[22,39], and decreased PTH secretion following $1,25(OH)_2D$ administration[17,40]. In addition, $1,25(OH)_2D$ increases gut transport of calcium[18,19].

The concept that resistance to the calcaemic effect of PTH occurs in azòtaemia was suggested by Stanbury and Lumb[41]. Subsequently, Massry and others have shown that patients with various degrees of renal insufficiency have a decreased calcaemic response to exogenous PTH[42]. The calcaemic response to endogenous PTH is also reduced in patients with early renal failure during hypocalcaemia induced by ethylenediamine-tetra-acetate (EDTA)[21]. In the experimental animal, the exogenous administration of 1,25$(OH)_2$D partially corrects the decreased calcaemic response to PTH[39]. In addition, phosphate restriction in early renal failure results in an increase in 1,25$(OH)_2$D levels, a decrease in PTH levels, and an improved calcaemic response to exogenously administered PTH[14]. Finally, we have shown that the administration of 0.25 μg 1,25$(OH)_2$D twice daily to patients with early renal failure results in normalization of the serum levels of 1,25$(OH)_2$D, an improvement in the impaired calcaemic response to PTH, a decrease in the level of urinary cyclic AMP (a marker of PTH activity), and normalization of the renal handling of phosphate[22]. In Figures 4.1 and 4.2, the effect of EDTA on serum calcium and PTH is shown before and after therapy with 1,25$(OH)_2$D. Treatment with 1,25$(OH)_2$D reduces the EDTA-induced decline in serum calcium and improves the recovery in serum calcium despite comparable levels of PTH. Thus, in summary, a deficiency of 1,25$(OH)_2$D both in early and advanced renal failure may play an important role in the development of secondary hyperparathyroidism.

A direct effect of 1,25$(OH)_2$D on PTH secretion may also be an important factor, and may alter the set point of calcium for PTH secretion in renal failure[43]. The set point is defined as the concentration of calcium necessary to produce a 50% decrease in PTH secretion. In addition, it has been shown that in renal failure adenylate cyclase of hyperplastic parathyroid glands is less susceptible to inhibition by calcium[44]. Previous studies have demonstrated an *in vivo* inhibitory effect of 1,25$(OH)_2$D on PTH release in the rat[45], and also an *in vitro* inhibitory effect on monolayer cell cultures of bovine parathyroid cells[15,46]. Other studies have shown specific binding of 1,25$(OH)_2$D to parathyroid tissue[47,48]. Both *in vitro* and *in vivo* studies have demonstrated that 1,25$(OH)_2$D decreases levels of preproparathyroid hormone messenger RNA[16,49]. These results suggest that 1,25$(OH)_2$D regulates PTH gene transcription. Finally, a recent study in dogs has shown that increased PTH levels developed during surgically induced renal failure despite the fact that the serum calcium was maintained above normal[17]. This was associated with a significant decrease in 1,25$(OH)_2$D levels. The administration of 1,25$(OH)_2$D to achieve normal levels prevented the increase of PTH, even in the absence of

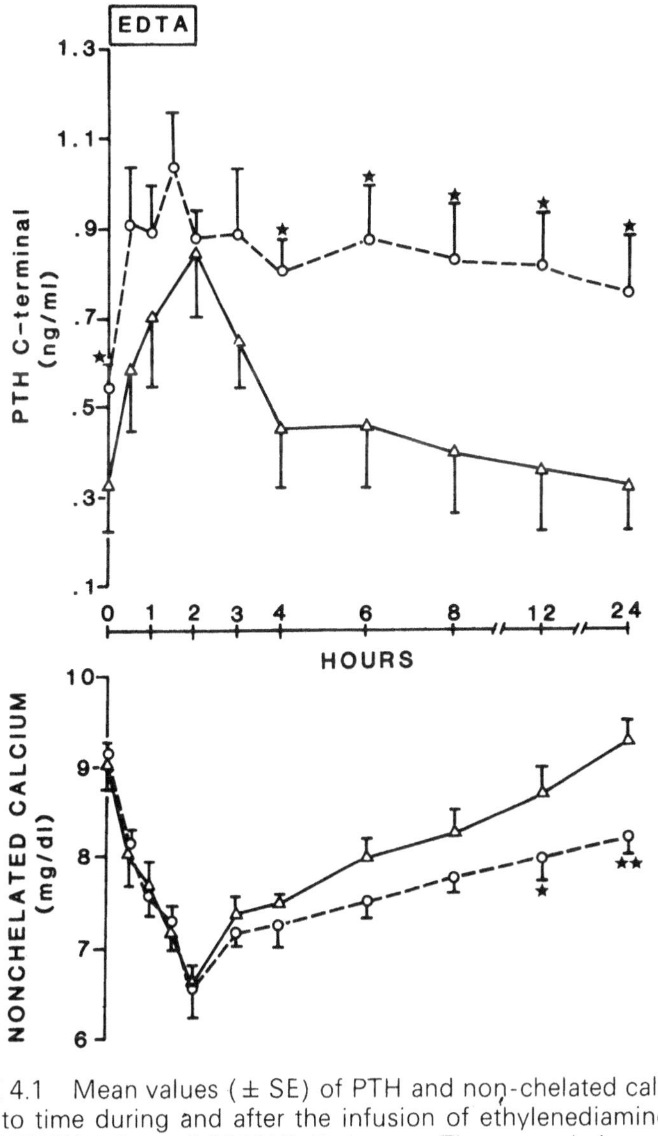

FIGURE 4.1 Mean values (± SE) of PTH and non-chelated calcium in relation to time during and after the infusion of ethylenediamine-tetra-acetate (EDTA) prior to $1{,}25(OH)_2D$ therapy. The open circles represent values from patients with early renal failure. The open triangles represent values from normal subjects. Symbols are: *, $p<0.05$; **, $p<0.01$. (From Wilson *et al.* (1985). *Kidney Int.*, **27,** 565–73; reproduced with permission)

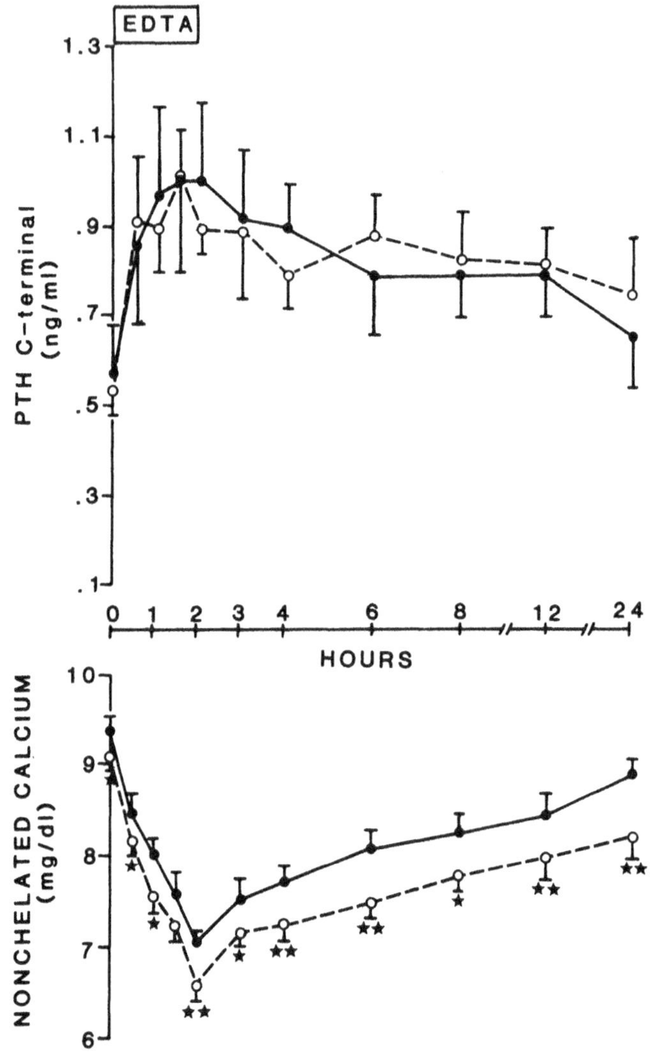

FIGURE 4.2 Mean values (± SE) of PTH and non-chelated calcium during the EDTA test in patients before (open circles) and after (closed circles) $1,25(OH)_2D$ therapy. Symbols are: *, $p<0.05$; **, $p<0.01$. (From Wilson *et al.* (1985). *Kidney Int.*, **27**, 565–73; reproduced with permission)

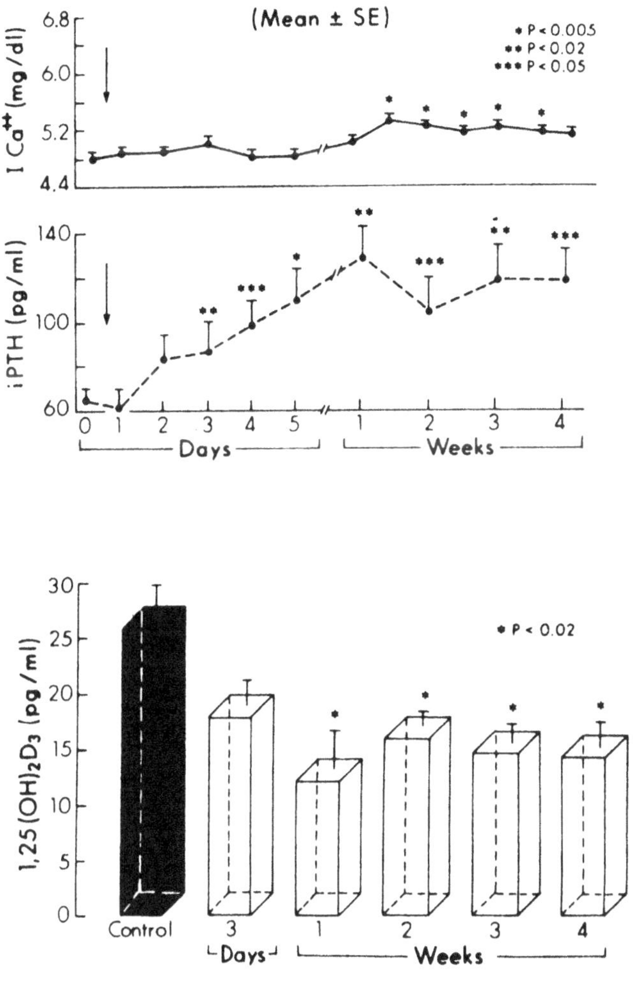

FIGURE 4.3 Serum-ionized calcium, amino iPTH levels, and serum $1,25(OH)_2D_3$ before and after the induction of renal insufficiency (arrow) in a group of six dogs from protocol I. ICa, ionized calcium. (From Lopez-Hilker *et al.* (1986). *J. Clin. Invest.*, **78,** 1097–102; reproduced with permission)

increased serum calcium (Figures 4.3 and 4.4). However, also of interest is that mild hypercalcaemia and high $1,25(OH)_2D$ levels did not result in undetectable levels of PTH[17]. Thus in summary, the above findings suggest that hypocalcaemia may not be the only factor

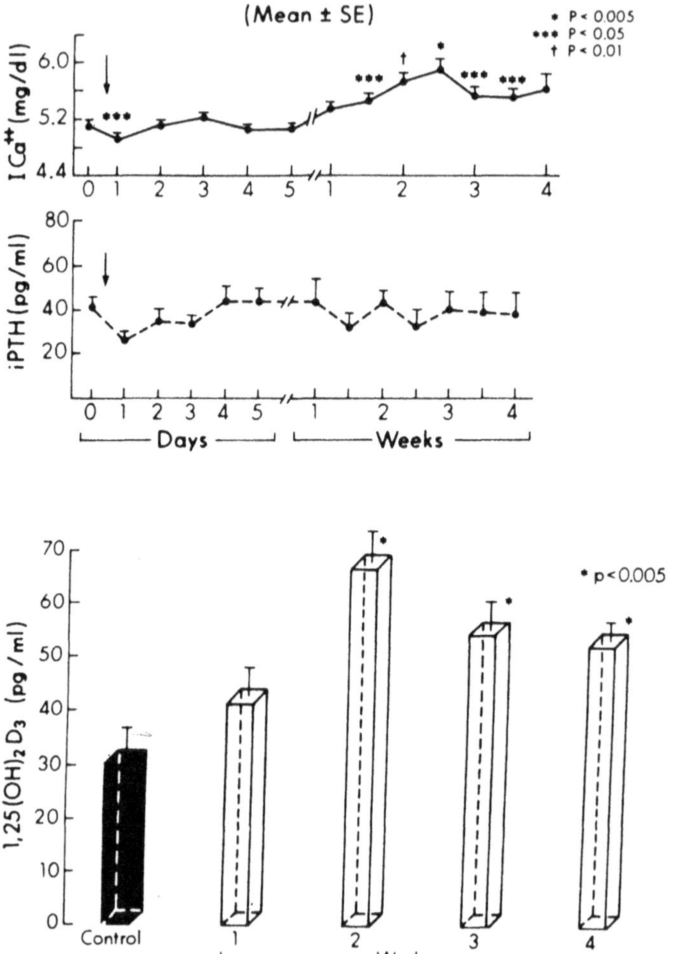

FIGURE 4.4 Serum-ionized calcium, amino iPTH levels and serum $1,25(OH)_2D_3$ in a group of five dogs from protocol II who received 150–200 ng of $1,25(OH)_2D_3$ twice daily, before and after the induction of renal insufficiency (arrow). ICa, ionized calcium. (From Lopez-Hilker *et al.* (1986). *J. Clin. Invest.*, **78,** 1097–102; reproduced with permission)

producing hyperparathyroidism in renal failure, and a deficiency of $1,25(OH)_2D$ may directly contribute to the development of hyperparathyroidism in chronic renal failure.

With advanced renal failure there is decreased gut calcium absorption[20], which is associated with decreased $1,25(OH)_2D$ levels. This defect is corrected with exogenous $1,25(OH)_2D$ administration[18,19]. In early renal failure, phosphate restriction will increase levels of $1,25(OH)_2D$ and correct the calcium malabsorption[21]. Thus, a deficiency of $1,25(OH)_2D$ produces calcium malabsorption and as a result contributes to the development of hypocalcaemia, a major factor in the production of hyperparathyroidism.

From the above discussion, it would appear that both hyperparathyroidism and a deficiency of $1,25(OH)_2D$ are important manifestations of early and advanced renal failure. The secondary hyperparathyroidism and the $1,25(OH)_2D$ deficiency are the primary factors responsible for the development of the bone disease, osteitis fibrosa. Other factors which may contribute to the development of osteitis fibrosa include abnormal collagen synthesis[50] and abnormal crystal growth and maturation[51,52].

BONE DISEASE

Before discussion of the various bone lesions observed in renal failure, a brief review of the bone structure is necessary. Indigenous to bone are three cell types - the osteoblast, the osteocyte and the osteoclast. The osteoblast deposits osteoid (unmineralized bone matrix). During active osteoid deposition, the osteoblast assumes a cuboidal or columnar shape and as the rate of matrix synthesis decreases, the osteoblast becomes progressively attenuated. As the osteoblast deposits osteoid, a few of these cells are incorporated in the osteoid, and with mineralization of the osteoid, become osteocytes within the mineralized bone. The osteocyte with its system of canaliculi (canals) covers a large surface area. The osteocyte may also change size in response to PTH. However, whether the osteocyte is capable of bone resorption remains a subject of controversy. It is difficult to conceive of a cell, whose initial function was bone formation, that could become responsible for bone resorption. The size changes, observed in osteocytes, may be secondary to the action of PTH on osteoblasts[53]. Osteoclasts are large, mobile multinucleated cells responsible for bone resorption. Their derivation is probably from monocyte–macrophage precursors[54]. Osteoclasts attach to non-osteoid bone surfaces and resorb bone. In general, there is a balance between bone formation and resorption. In the young individual, the balance favours formation and accumulation of bone, while after the third or fourth decade, the balance favours resorption and loss of bone. In this process of bone formation and resorption, bone acts as a repository and source of calcium. However, this function of bone is beyond the scope of this chapter, and is reviewed elsewhere[55, 56].

The natural sequence of bone formation includes osteoid deposition followed by mineralization. The biochemical process of mineralization, involving changes from amorphous calcium phosphate to calcium hydroxyapatite, is not well understood. The antibiotic, tetracycline, can be used as a marker of bone mineralization. Tetracycline binds to newly deposited bone mineral and when bone is viewed with fluorescent light, the tetracycline will fluoresce[57]. Consequently, if two separate doses of tetracycline are given, for example 10 days apart, then the distance between tetracycline labels divided by the number of days between doses will provide the rate of mineralization. The rate of mineralization times the fraction of mineralized surface provides the bone formation rate.

In reality, renal osteodystrophy includes various bone lesions. These have been divided into four categories: (1) osteitis fibrosa, (2) mixed osteitis fibrosa–osteomalacia, (3) 'low turnover' osteomalacia (LTOM), and (4) aplastic bone disease. Osteitis fibrosa is characterized by a marked increase in osteoblasts and osteoclasts, the presence of bone marrow fibrosis (termed endosteal fibrosis), and an increase in the bone formation rate. A characteristic example of osteitis fibrosa is shown in Figures 4.5 and 4.6. Mixed osteitis fibrosa–osteomalacia has features of both osteitis fibrosa and osteomalacia. These include increased cellular activity, some endosteal fibrosis, abnormally wide osteoid seams, and a bone formation rate that is active but below the expected rate for the degree of cellular activity. Often the distance between the two tetracycline labels is not well separated. An example is shown in Figures 4.7 and 4.8. Low turnover osteomalacia is characterized by a marked reduction in cellular activity, broad osteoid seams, and the complete or almost complete cessation of bone formation. In more than 90% of these cases, histological staining of aluminium is found. Characteristic bone histological findings of LTOM are shown in Figures 4.9 and 4.10. Finally, the least common of the

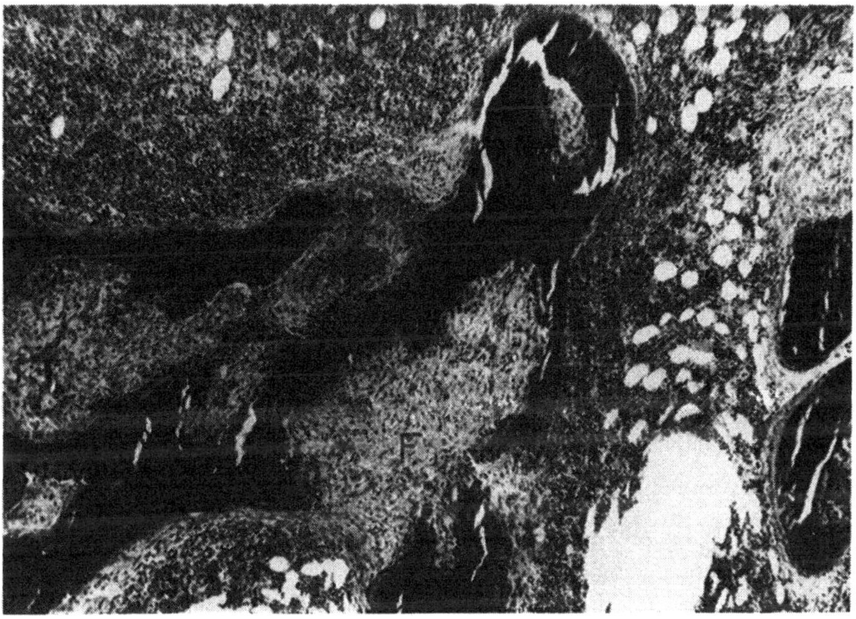

FIGURE 4.5 An example of osteitis fibrosa is shown. The presence of endosteal fibrosis (F) and increased cellular activity is apparent (× 87)

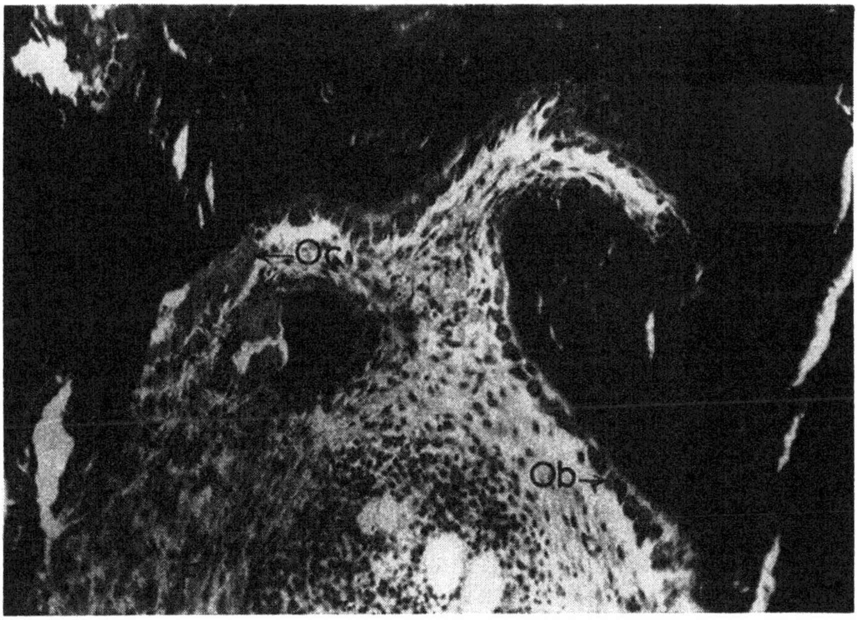

FIGURE 4.6 Endosteal fibrosis (F), osteoblasts (Ob), and osteoclasts (Oc) are observed in this example of osteitis fibrosa (× 140)

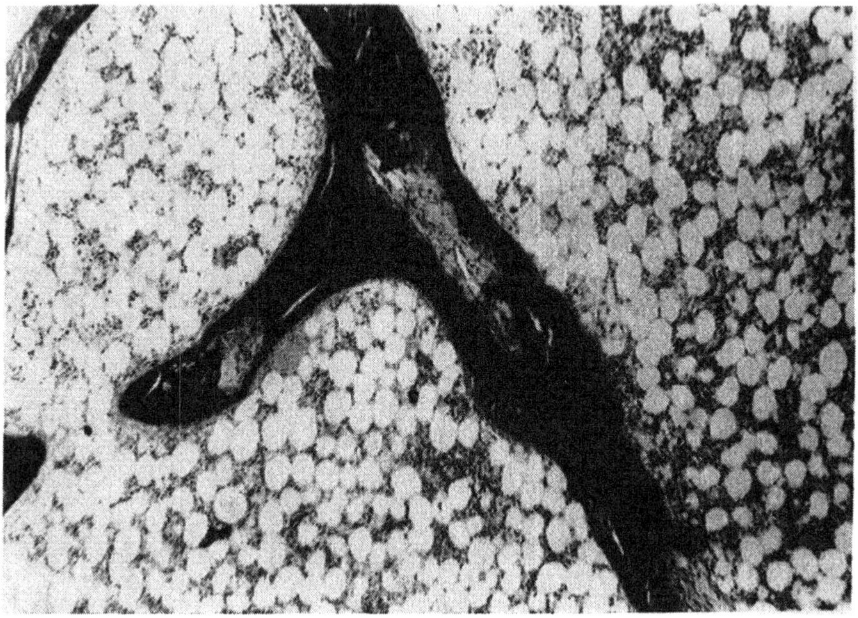

FIGURE 4.7 An example of mixed osteitis fibrosa–osteomalacia is shown (× 87)

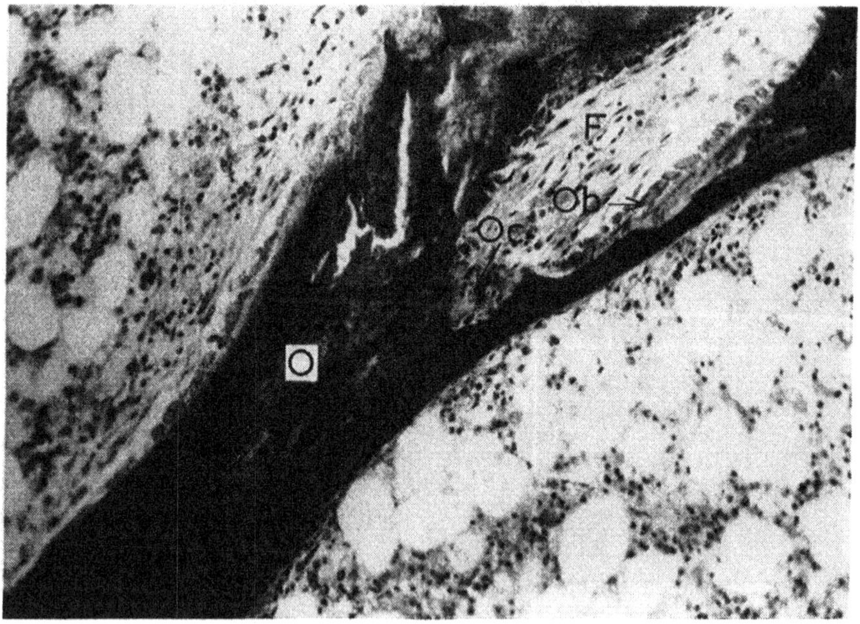

FIGURE 4.8 At higher magnification, increased cellular activity, osteoblasts (Ob) and osteoclasts (Oc), and endosteal fibrosis (F) are observed. However, at the same time, large osteoid deposits (O) are present (× 140)

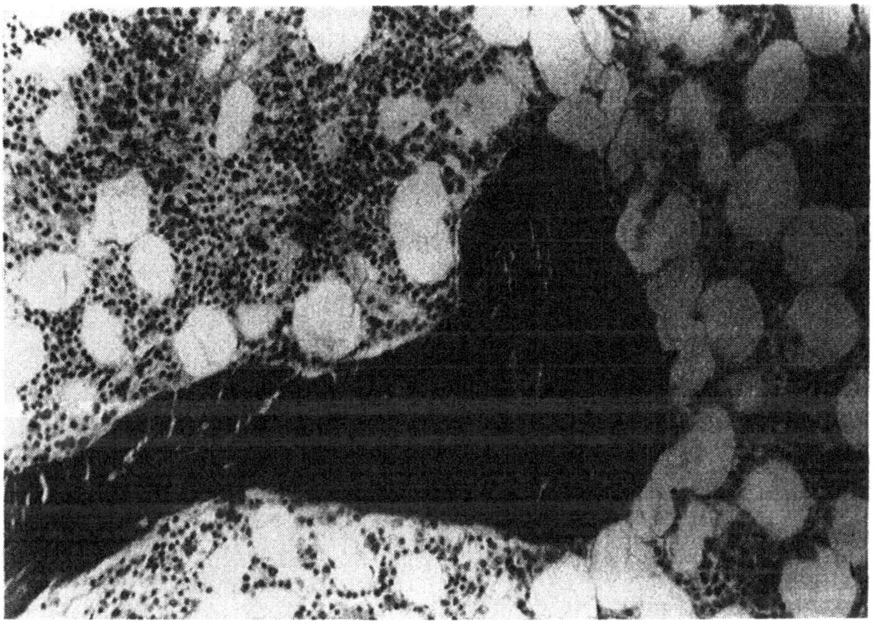

FIGURE 4.9 An example of low turnover osteomalacia is shown. The findings are characterized by large osteoid deposits (O) and the absence of cellular activity and endosteal fibrosis (× 140)

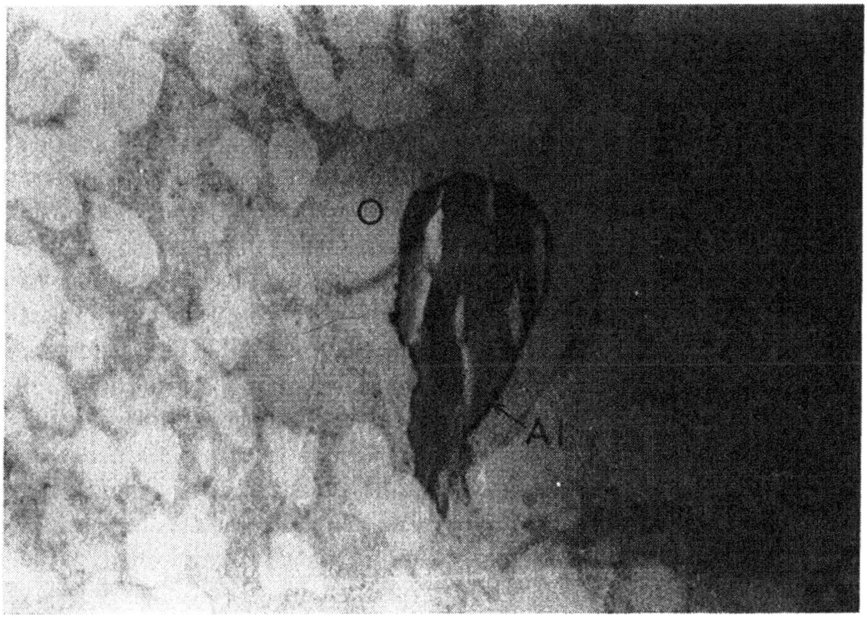

FIGURE 4.10 An example of aluminium deposits is shown. The aluminium (Al) is present at the interface of osteoid (O) and mineralized bone (× 140)

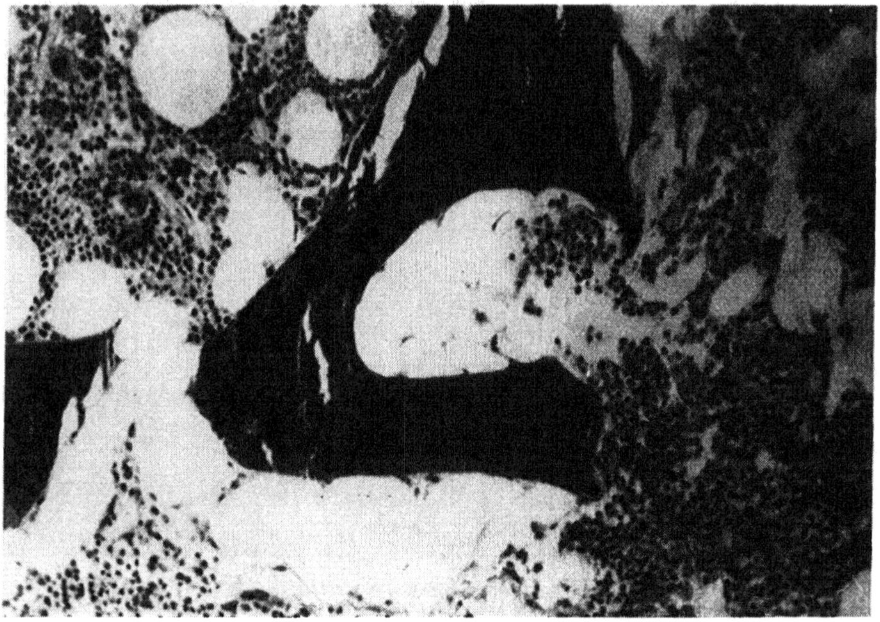

FIGURE 4.11 Aplastic bone disease is characterized by the absence of cellular activity, endosteal fibrosis and large osteoid deposits ($\times 140$)

four categories is aplastic bone disease. Similar to LTOM, features include minimal cellular activity and the virtual cessation of bone formation. However, there is no accumulation of osteoid and positive aluminium staining is not found as often and generally is not as dense. An example of aplastic bone disease is shown in Figure 4.11.

The development of osteitis fibrosa is presumed to be secondary to very high levels of PTH. Indeed when PTH levels have been compared to histological criteria of increased bone turnover, PTH levels are very high in osteitis fibrosa[58–62]. However, there are a vast multitude of clinically available PTH assays and PTH levels are generally increased in renal failure[63]. Thus, for the best results a comparison of the PTH assay and bone histology should be available. An elevated PTH concentration may not be sufficient to diagnose osteitis fibrosa. In some PTH assays a three-fold elevation of PTH may suggest the presence of osteitis fibrosa, while in others a 30–50-fold increase may be indicative of severe secondary hyperparathyroidism.

In patients with early to advanced renal failure or receiving maintenance dialysis, osteitis fibrosa is the predominant finding[64,65]. In addition to osteitis fibrosa, mixed osteitis fibrosa–osteomalacia may be considered in this category since levels of PTH are also elevated. In a previous study we evaluated 142 unselected maintenance dialysis patients from a single geographic region[65]. Both osteitis fibrosa and osteitis fibrosa–osteomalacia were categorized as osteitis fibrosa. Of the 142 haemodialysed patients, 96 (68%) had osteitis fibrosa. As shown in Table 4.1, clinically apparent musculoskeletal problems were not common in this group. Biochemically, as shown in Figures 4.12 and 4.13, the serum calcium was significantly lower in osteitis fibrosa than LTOM ($p<0.05$), and serum alkaline phosphatase was increased compared with both LTOM and aplastic bone disease ($p<0.05$); no significant differences were present in serum phosphorus. In addition, the carboxy terminal PTH level was higher ($p<0.01$) and the serum aluminium lower ($p<0.05$) in osteitis fibrosa than the other two groups.

The criteria selected for the histological diagnosis by definition lead to significant differences in bone histomorphometric parameters between the three groups. Thus statistical analysis was not performed, but nevertheless, the magnitude of these differences is important to appreciate and consequently they are presented in Figure 4.14. Osteoblasts, osteoclasts and endosteal fibrosis are markedly increased in osteitis fibrosis. Of interest to note are the minimal differences in total osteoid surface and relative osteoid volume between osteitis fibrosa and LTOM. The expectation is that LTOM would have a large accumulation of osteoid. However, in osteitis fibrosa the amount of osteoid accumulation is defined by the equilibrium between osteoid

TABLE 4.1 Initial clinical findings in 142 haemodialysis patients

	Muscle weakness	*Bone pain*	*Fractures*
Osteitis fibrosa (*N*=96)	5 (5%)	4 (4%)	3 (3%)
Osteomalacia (*N*=36)	15 (40%)	13 (35%)	10 (27%)
Aplastic bone disease (*N*=10)	2 (20%)	3 (30%)	2 (20%)

From Llach *et al.* (1986). *Kidney Int.*, **29** (Suppl. 18), S74–9, reproduced with permission

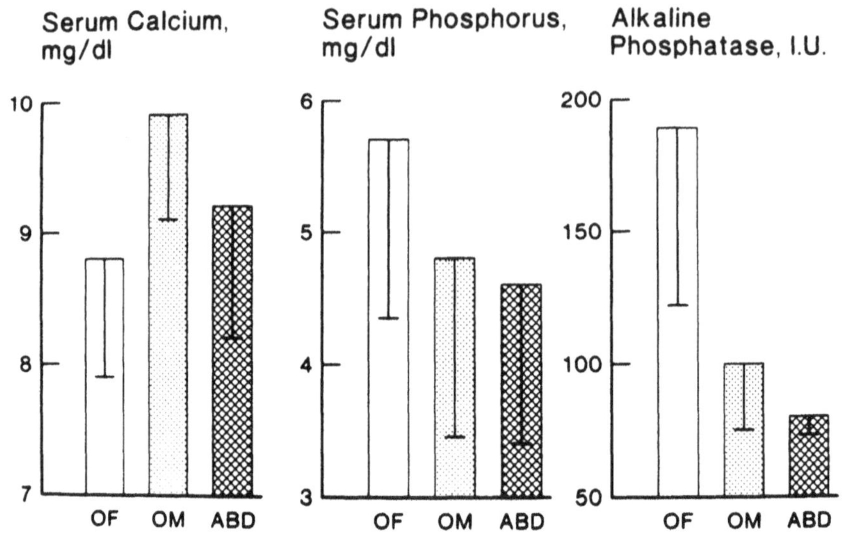

FIGURE 4.12 Mean (±SD) serum calcium and phosphorus concentrations and alkaline phosphatase activity in dialysis patients with osteitis fibrosa (OF), osteomalacia (OM), and aplastic bone disease (ABD); normal alkaline phosphatase, 30–100 Iu/l. (From Llach *et al.* (1986). *Kidney Int.*, **29** (Suppl. 18), S74–9; reproduced with permission)

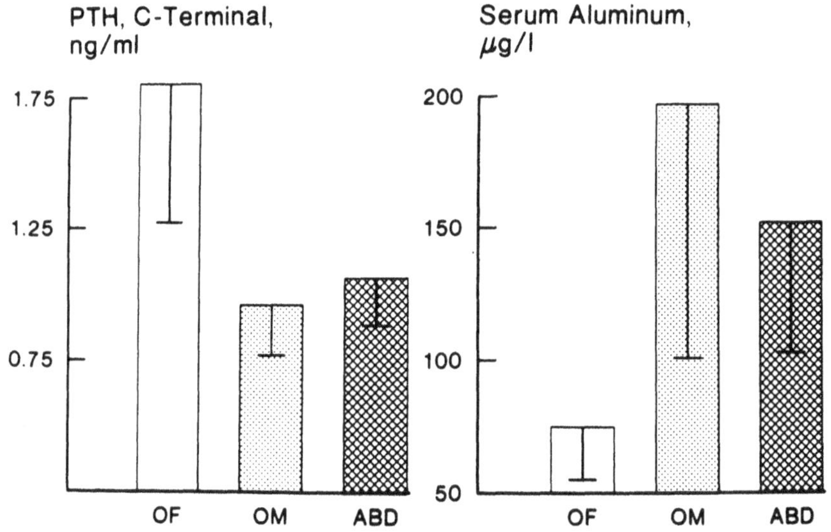

FIGURE 4.13 Mean (±SD) parathyroid hormone levels and aluminium concentration in patients with osteitis fibrosa (OF), osteomalacia (OM), and aplastic bone disease (ABD). Normal range for PTH, 0.1–0.3 ng/ml; aluminium, 2.3–6.4 g/l. (From Llach *et al.* (1986). *Kidney Int.*, **29** (Suppl. 18), S74–9; reproduced with permission)

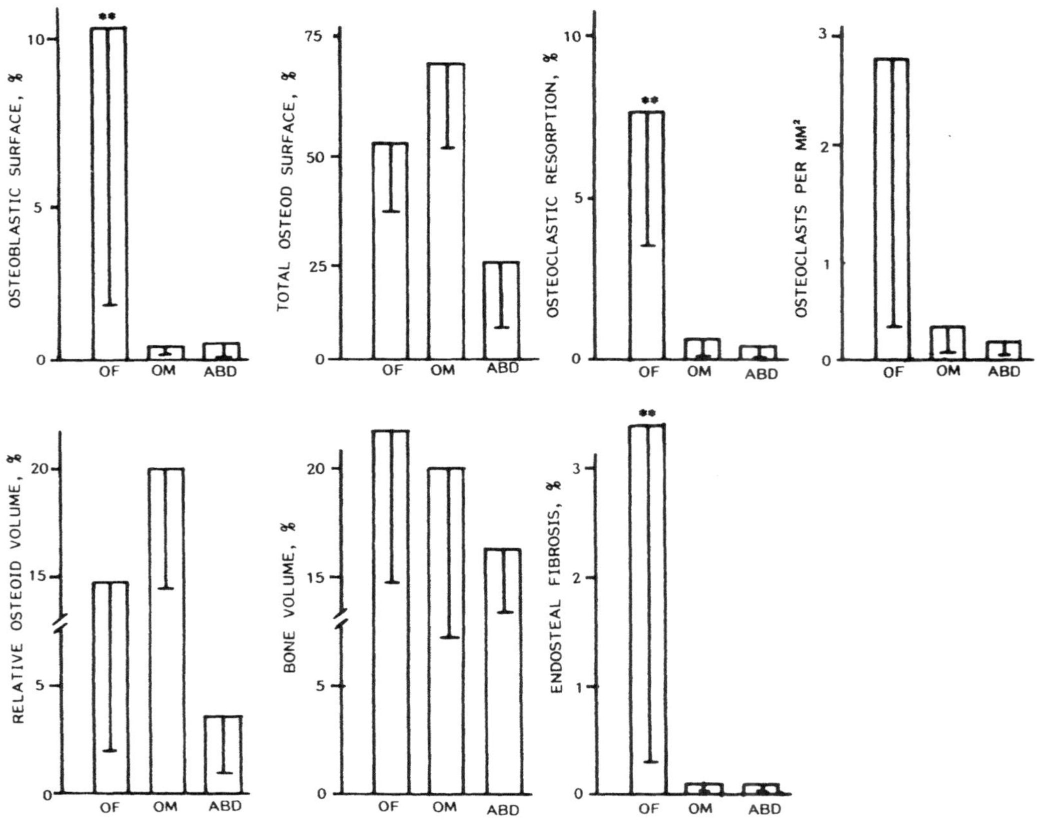

FIGURE 4.14 Bone histomorphometric findings (±SD) in patients with osteitis fibrosa (OF), osteomalacia (OM), and aplastic bone disease (ABD). (From Llach *et al.* (1986). *Kidney Int.*, **29** (Suppl. 18), S74–9; reproduced with permission)

deposition and the rate of bone formation. Thus, even if bone formation is normal or exceeds normal, osteoid will accumulate if osteoid deposition is greater than the rate mineralized bone is formed. Thus, as opposed to LTOM in which both the rate of osteoid deposition and bone mineralization are reduced, osteoid accumulation in both osteitis fibrosa and mixed disease is secondary to a different dynamic equilibrium. In this instance, an increased rate of osteoid deposition exceeds a bone formation rate that ranges from minimally decreased to greater than normal.

While the evolution of osteitis fibrosa and mixed disease can be understood on an aetiological basis, factors leading to the development of LTOM are more difficult to understand. Initially, it was assumed that osteomalacia resulted from a deficiency of $1,25(OH)_2D$, a known consequence of renal failure. However, more than a decade ago, it was shown that even in anephric patients, a group expected to have minimal if any circulating $1,25(OH)_2D$, the predominant histological lesion was osteitis fibrosa[66]. Subsequently, when $1,25(OH)_2D$ became available for clinical studies, it was demonstrated that $1,25(OH)_2D$ failed to improve LTOM[67,68]. However, $1,25(OH)_2D$ did prove to be of value in treatment of mixed osteitis fibrosa–osteomalacia[69,70]. Thus, it became apparent that LTOM was not due to a deficiency of $1,25(OH)_2D$. Subsequent studies during the past 10 years have demonstrated an association between aluminium and LTOM. Several lines of study suggest the aetiological role of aluminium in the pathogenesis of LTOM. Thus, epidemiological studies in Great Britain documented a regional clustering of cases with LTOM[71]. Subsequently, LTOM was associated with the presence of aluminium in the dialysis water[72–74]. In addition, investigation in animals showed that aluminium administration produced osteomalacia[75,76]. A rediscovery of an older histological stain has documented the presence of aluminium along the trabecular surface, at the interface of osteoid and mineralized bone, and in reversal lines (the sites of old resorption cavities which have been filled with mineralized bone)[77]. Finally, the administration of the chelating agent, desferrioxamine, has improved bone histology and reduced the aluminium burden[78,79]. All of these findings have strongly implicated aluminium as the cause of LTOM.

The clinical presentation of LTOM often includes a tendency to develop hypercalcaemia, diffuse musculoskeletal pain, fractures, and a relative deficiency of PTH[65,67]. The tendency to develop hypercalcaemia is an interesting finding. As is seen in Figure 4.12, it is often present even in the absence of treatment with vitamin D metabolites, and marked hypercalcaemia may result during treatment with vitamin D metabolites or analogues[67]. The cause of the hypercalcaemia is postulated to be the failure to move calcium into bone[80]. Since in LTOM there is a virtual cessation of bone formation, and with renal failure, the kidney cannot excrete calcium, any stimulus for increased gut calcium absorption or the use of increased dialysate calcium may lead to hypercalcaemia. Similar findings have been observed in aluminium loaded animals[81–84].

As is observed in Figure 4.13, a relative PTH deficiency is present in LTOM. The term, relative, is used because the PTH level is usually above the normal range (due to the presence of renal failure), but lower than that observed in patients with osteitis fibrosa. In the past, the obvious question was whether the relative deficiency of PTH was secondary to the hypercalcaemia. However, studies addressing this question by producing hypocalcaemia with a calcium-free dialysis demonstrated that hypocalcaemia failed to elicit an appropriate PTH response[85,86]. Data from our laboratory showing such a response are displayed in Figure 4.15. Such findings suggested the possibility that aluminium may directly inhibit PTH secretion. Several tissue culture studies have indicated that aluminium does inhibit PTH secretion[87,88]. The relative PTH deficiency may be important in the development of LTOM, since PTH may protect against the toxic effects of aluminium on bone[89,90].

Musculoskeletal pain and fractures are common clinical features of LTOM. For several years it was believed that these findings were observed in all patients with LTOM since the majority of bone biopsies obtained in symptomatic patients revealed LTOM[67]. However, recently we have shown in a prospective study (Table 4.1) that although fractures and musculoskeletal pain are more common in LTOM, these occurred in less than one half of patients[65]. As shown in Table 4.2, when these same patients were followed for 2 years, the incidence of bone pain, muscle weakness and fractures increased markedly. This occurred despite no significant change in serum calcium, phosphorus, alkaline phosphatase and PTH. Furthermore, a high mortality rate was observed in this group of 36 patients. Thirteen

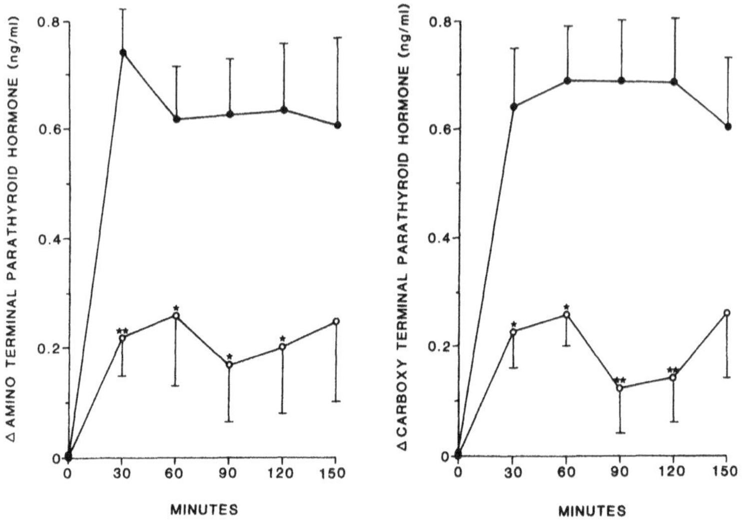

FIGURE 4.15 A comparison of PTH response to hypocalcaemia in osteomalacia (O) and osteitis fibrosa (●). The amino terminal PTH response was significantly greater at 30, 60, 90 and 120 min in osteitis fibrosa. $^*p<0.05$; ** $p<0.01$. The carboxy terminal PTH response was significantly greater at 30, 60, 90 and 120 min in osteitis fibrosa. $^*p<0.05$; ** $p<0.01$. (From Andress *et al.* (1983). *Kidney Int.*, **24**, 364–70; reproduced with permission)

of the 36 patients died during the 2-year period of observation. Causes of death included congestive heart failure (8), sepsis (3), CNS (? dialysis dementia) (1), and discontinuation of haemodialysis because of patient's request (1). The development of musculoskeletal symptoms appeared to herald the onset of an increased mortality rate[65].

Aplastic bone disease was observed in 7% of our 142 maintenance

TABLE 4.2 Clinical findings in 36 patients with osteomalacia

	Muscle weakness	*Bone pain*	*Fractures*
At time of biopsy	15 (42%)	13 (36%)	10(28%)
At end of study	24 (67%)	22 (61%)	15 (42%)

From Llach *et al.* (1986). *Kidney Int.*, **29** (Suppl. 18), S74–9, reproduced with permission

haemodialysis patients. As can be observed from Table 4.1, clinical symptomatology was similar to the group with LTOM. Similar to LTOM (Figures 4.12 and 4.13), serum alkaline phosphatase and PTH levels were decreased compared to osteitis fibrosa ($p<0.05$). Serum aluminium was elevated in aplastic bone disease compared to osteitis fibrosa ($p<0.05$). As shown in Figure 4.14, the bone histology of aplastic bone disease resembles LTOM except that osteoid deposits are markedly reduced. Aluminium deposits were present in the majority of patients with aplastic bone disease[65]. Others have reported similar findings[91]. The question remains whether aplastic bone disease is the result of aluminium toxicity, and if so, why are the large osteoid deposits not present? In a preliminary study, we have shown that the administration of aluminium to parathyroidectomized rats with renal failure results in a histological entity resembling aplastic bone disease. If aluminium is administered to a parathyroid intact rat with renal failure, the histological findings are similar to LTOM[82]. This study suggests that the degree of parathyroid activity may be a moderator of the aluminium effect on bone.

The definitive diagnosis of renal osteodystrophy requires a bone biopsy, most accessible from the anterior iliac crest. Attempts have been made to diagnose renal osteodystrophy by non-invasive means. The two primary diagnostic tests employed are serum biochemistry and radiography. While both do provide valuable information, a specific diagnosis of the type of bone disease is often difficult to achieve.

Serum chemistries often provide useful information, but there is considerable overlap with the various histological lesions. In general, the serum calcium and phosphorus are of little diagnostic value. Hypercalcaemia and hyperphosphataemia occur frequently in severe osteitis fibrosa, but are also common in LTOM[65,92–94]. The reasons for the development of hypercalcaemia and hyperphosphataemia in these two disorders are probably different. In severe osteitis fibrosa, accelerated removal of calcium and phosphorus from bone probably accounts for the hypercalcaemia and hyperphosphataemia. In LTOM, the most likely reason is the inability to deposit calcium and phosphorus in bone. Serum PTH is often helpful as a diagnostic test. As mentioned previously, a knowledge of the correlation of the specific PTH assay with bone histology, and an appreciation of the range of changes in PTH levels in renal failure are important. We, as well as other investigators, have reported a correlation between serum PTH and the magnitude of bone activity. Thus, although PTH levels are, in general, highest in severe osteitis fibrosa and lowest in LTOM[60, 62, 85, 86], considerable overlap does exist in the various forms of renal osteodystrophy. Significant correlation also has been reported between serum alkaline phosphatase and bone activity[59, 65, 92, 95]. The elevation in serum alkaline phosphatase is presumed secondary to osteoblastic activity. In the epidemic forms of LTOM reported in Great Britain during the 1970s, the serum alkaline phosphatase level was generally in the normal range and thus, clearly different from the increased levels observed in osteitis fibrosa[67, 92, 96, 97]. However, in the more sporadic cases of LTOM, the serum alkaline phosphatase concentration is often moderately elevated. Thus, serum alkaline phosphatase is probably not as discriminating as would be desired. In addition, elevations in serum PTH and alkaline phosphatase do not exclude the presence of aluminium. Recently, studies have been performed with Gla-protein, also known as osteocalcin, the most abundant non-collagenous protein in bone. Circulating Gla-protein levels generally reflect bone formation. In one study, a marked increase was present in osteitis fibrosa as compared to LTOM[98]. In general, the experience with Gla-protein is not very extensive, and in addition multiple forms may be present in uraemic serum[99]. Thus, more data are required to evaluate its usefulness.

The second major non-invasive technique for the assessment of renal osteodystrophy is radiography. Useful information can be gained from skeletal radiography if the proper techniques are applied. Magnification radiography of the hand bones with fine grain industrial film is the most advantageous technique[100–102]. Subperiosteal resorption is probably the earliest manifestation of overt secondary hyperparathyroidism and is best observed at the middle phalangeal radial surfaces or terminal phalangeal tufts[102, 103]. Several studies have shown positive correlations with microscopic grading of periosteal resorption and the severity of osteitis fibrosa[59, 103, 104]. However, the technique may not be sensitive enough. In one study, 38 of 58 patients with bone histological features of hyperparathyroidism had no subperiosteal resorption[93]. In other studies, subperiosteal resorption has been found in less than 50% of patients with osteitis fibrosa[92, 103]. Another complicating factor concerns false positive findings in patients with LTOM. As is apparent from bone histology, old resorption cavities are filled with osteoid. Since osteoid is radiolucent, the radiograph has the appearance of active bone resorption and may be incorrectly diagnosed as osteitis fibrosa[105]. Radiographic techniques capable of detecting osteomalacia are in general less sensitive[106].

In one recent study, the ^{99m}technetium-labelled methylene diphosphonate bone scan was used to evaluate renal osteodystrophy[107]. This technique was able to differentiate between LTOM and osteitis fibrosa, but overlap existed with mixed osteitis fibrosa–osteomalacia. However, other investigators have concluded that the bone scan did not provide useful information in the diagnosis of renal osteodystrophy[108].

While the radiographic tests reported above may be helpful, the principal diagnostic tool for renal osteodystrophy remains the bone biopsy and the processing of the undecalcified bone. From the histological preparation of bone, the extent of cellular activity, amount of osteoid, presence of endosteal fibrosis, bone mineralization and formation as evaluated by tetracycline labelling, and presence of aluminium can all be learned from the direct examination of bone. Aluminium is almost uniformly present in LTOM, frequently in aplastic disease, and also may be present in mixed osteitis fibrosa–osteomalacia; it is infrequently observed in osteitis fibrosa.

Extraosseous calcifications are frequently observed in uraemia and are a complex issue. Three principal forms of extraosseous calcification are found in uraemia. These include (1) calcification of medium-size arteries, (2) periarticular or tumoral calcifications, and (3) visceral calcifications affecting the heart, lung and kidneys[106]. A particularly severe form of metastatic calcification is the syndrome of calciphylaxis in which extensive vascular calcifications result in rapid development of skin ulcers[109]. The syndrome of calciphylaxis is a medical emergency and often responds to parathyroidectomy[109]. A review of the cellular basis of pathologic calcification is beyond the scope of this chapter, but is important to the understanding of the metastatic calcification process in uraemia and can be found elsewhere[110].

The reasons for calcification and the types of calcification may differ with location. Investigators have found that the visceral calcifications are amorphous calcium phosphate while arterial and non-visceral calcifications are hydroxyapatite[111,112]. Arterial calcifications are common in dialysis patients and are probably responsible for the high cardiovascular mortality of these patients[113]. Arterial calcifications can also result in pseudohypertension[114]. Visceral calcifications infrequently produce clinically apparent disease, but restrictive and diffusion pulmonary defects and heart block have been reported[115,116]. The pathogenesis of the extraosseous calcifications may differ. The calcium phosphate product is probably important in periarticular and tumoral calcifications[117], but an excess of PTH also may play a role[118]. In vascular and visceral calcifications, the role of the calcium phosphate product and PTH is not clear. However, studies in animals with renal failure have demonstrated that parathyroidectomy prevented the development of arterial calcifications and cardiac calcium accumulation[119,120].

Studies concerning the effect of continuous ambulatory peritoneal dialysis (CAPD) on renal osteodystrophy are inconclusive. In some studies vitamin D metabolites or analogues were administered[121,122], and in others oral calcium supplements were given[123,124]. In addition CAPD has resulted in decreased 25 hydroxyvitamin D levels[121,123,125]. Furthermore, most of the studies have included both patients with osteitis fibrosa and LTOM[121–126]. It would appear that osteitis fibrosa progresses during CAPD unless oral calcium supplementation and possibly vitamin D analogues or metabolites are administered[125,126]. Less convincing evidence suggests that LTOM may improve with CAPD[124,126].

Successful renal transplantation is the goal of most maintenance dialysis programmes. While a successful renal transplant markedly improves the well-being of the patient, skeletal problems, both new and residual, are often encountered. With transplantation, endogenous 1,25 dihydroxyvitamin D levels increase[127,128] and the hyperphosphataemia is corrected[129–132]. Residual hyperparathyroidism is a frequent problem and may lead to hypercalcaemia[129,132]. As long as the serum calcium remains less than 3 mmol/l (12 mg/dl), the function of the transplanted kidney is rarely impaired and parathyroidectomy is not advisable[129,131]. The hypophosphataemia often present may be secondary to either residual hyperparathyroidism[133,134] or primary phosphate loss by the transplanted kidney[134,135]. Finally, corticosteroids, used as immunosuppressive agents, may result in loss of bone mass.

For the most part, clinically apparent skeletal problems are infrequent with successful renal transplantation. Osteitis fibrosa generally improves, but increased bone cellular activity often never completely resolves; long-term hyperparathyroidism may be present because of incomplete involution of the parathyroid gland[132,136] or because the continued mild-to-moderate decrement of GFR remains a stimulus for PTH secretion[7,8,17]. Available information on the effect of renal transplantation on LTOM is minimal, but case reports do indicate improvement[137,138]. However, desferrioxamine may also have to be used after transplantation[139]. It has been suggested that the hypophosphataemia may produce osteomalacia, and in one report osteomalacia was diagnosed by X-ray[140]. However, in a study of ten long-term hypophosphataemic renal transplant recipients, we did not observe osteomalacia in any patient[141]. The primary finding in these patients was a decrease in bone volume. However, some also had a decrease in bone formation rate but not a concomitant increase in osteoid.

The most disabling skeletal problem in the renal transplant recipient is the development of aseptic necrosis. The incidence of aseptic necrosis has varied from 3 to 41%[142–144]. The aetiology of aseptic necrosis remains unclear as is evident from the different names, avascular necrosis, osteonecrosis, ischaemic necrosis, given to the process. Extensive reviews of this problem have been published elsewhere[145–151]. Aseptic necrosis is not unique to renal transplantation and develops in other clinical conditions[145–151]. Postulated pathogenic mechanisms include (1) trabecular microfractures which develop due to the lack of bone remodelling – these subsequently accumulate and produce macroscopic fractures[152,153], (2) subchondral fractures through osteopenic bone which interrupt the blood supply[146], (3) cell death from cytotoxic factors[147,150,151], and (4) vascular causes[150,151]. Included in the vascular category are extraosseous arterial and venous causes such as arterial thrombosis and disease of the deep venous system; intraosseous arterial and venous disease which include microemboli, fat emboli or intravenous thrombosis, all of which may occlude the circulation; and, finally, intraosseous extravascular factors in which bone marrow pressures increase producing a compartmental syndrome. Bone marrow pressures are often elevated in aseptic necrosis, and results with simple decompression have been promising, especially when the aseptic necrosis is diagnosed at an early stage[149, 150].

The incidence of aseptic necrosis in renal transplant recipients varies according to whether the figures are based on all renal transplants or those surviving for at least 12 months. The onset of symptoms is often within the first year[144, 154, 155], and the most commonly involved joint is the femoral head[146, 154, 155]. However, primary involvement of other joints may be observed[144, 154, 155], and multiple involvement is not uncommon[144, 154, 155]. It has been difficult to extract predisposing factors in the majority of the published series. In some series, the steroid dose and the number of rejection episodes with high-dose steroids have been predictive factors[154, 156], but in most, the steroid dose has not[142, 144, 155, 157]. However, the very high doses of steroids employed during the early years of most renal transplantation programmes may have been a predisposing factor[144, 156]. At present early diagnosis is important because intervention at this stage may prevent the progession of the process[149, 150]. The traditional approach has been the X-ray, but the bone scan[158], magnetic resonance imaging[159], and single photon emission computed tomography[160] may be more sensitive.

TREATMENT

The approach to the treatment of the patient with renal osteodystrophy must be individualized. Effective therapy for osteitis fibrosa is generally ineffective treatment of LTOM. The presence of aluminium in a patient with severe osteitis fibrosa may dissuade the attending nephrologist from recommending parathyroidectomy. The finding of LTOM and aluminium may be an indication for a modification of the patient's antacid regimen. Treatment of hypercalcaemia in osteitis fibrosa and LTOM should be approached differently. Thus, knowledge of the pathological findings should modify the therapeutic approach to the patient.

Vitamin D metabolites and analogues have been used for the treatment of renal osteodystrophy. Vitamin D was used for treatment of renal osteodystrophy in 1927 by Parsons[2]. Unlike the dramatic response observed in vitamin D-dependent rickets and osteomalacia secondary to malabsorption, the hyperparathyroid bone disease of renal failure did not respond. Advances in vitamin D biochemistry resulted in discovery and availability of 25 hydroxyvitamin D and 1,25 dihydroxyvitamin D. Treatment with vitamin D has resulted in improvement of osteitis fibrosa[161, 162]. However, because of its long half-life and the availability of other more physiologically active metabolites and analogues, the use of vitamin D is not indicated for the treatment of renal osteodystrophy[163].

Dihydrotachysterol (DHT), a synthetic compound with a structure similar to $1,25(OH)_2D$, has been available since 1943[164]. The 'A ring' of DHT is rotated 180° with the hydroxyl group at carbon 3 occupying the stereochemical equivalent of the 1-hydroxyl group in $1,25(OH)_2D$[163]. After hepatic hydroxylation at the 25 position, DHT has a configuration similar to $1,25(OH)_2D$. DHT has been evaluated in a limited number of studies, and has, in general, produced symptomatic, radiographic and skeletal improvement in patients with both osteitis fibrosa and mixed osteitis fibrosa–osteomalacia[165, 166]. Since activation of DHT requires 25 hydroxylation, its effectiveness in patients with liver disease or patients receiving anticonvulsants may be decreased.

The intermediate metabolite, 25OHD, is produced by 25 hydroxylation of vitamin D by the liver. Plasma half-life is estimated to be 20–30 days[167]; thus, daily dosage is adequate. However, pharmacological doses of the drug and markedly elevated serum levels are necessary to achieve a therapeutic effect. Therapy with 25OHD increases gut absorption of calcium, decreases PTH, and improves the bone histology of osteitis fibrosa and mixed osteitis fibrosa–osteomalacia[168,169]. The decreased PTH levels are most probably secondary to increased serum calcium levels. As discussed previously, $1,25(OH)_2D$ directly binds to the parathyroid gland and inhibits PTH secretion; however, so far there is no evidence to suggest that 25OHD has a similar action.

Numerous clinical studies are available on the use of $1,25(OH)_2D$ and its synthetic analogue 1α-hydroxyvitamin D[170–174]. Both will be considered together. In general, the response to osteitis fibrosa and mixed osteitis fibrosa–osteomalacia has been favourable. Both bone pain and proximal muscle weakness have been reported to improve after $1,25(OH)_2D$[170–173]. Hypercalcaemia is a frequent problem with $1,25(OH)_2D$ and 1α-OHD therapy. Patients with mild baseline hypercalcaemia often become markedly hypercalcaemic during early therapy while those with hypocalcaemia generally become hypercalcaemic only after approximately 1 year of therapy[173, 175, 176]. In the latter instance, hypercalcaemia is generally not observed until the serum alkaline phosphatase approaches normal[177]. Provided that the bone biopsy has eliminated the possibility of LTOM, the majority of the patients with early hypercalcaemia have severe osteitis fibrosa. They may require a parathyroidectomy for control of overt hyperparathyroidism. Most episodes of 1,25$(OH)_2$D-induced hypercalcaemia are mild and asymptomatic, and will resolve within 2–5 days after discontinuation of 1,25$(OH)_2D_3$.

Serum alkaline phosphatase and PTH levels decrease as a result of treatment with 1,25$(OH)_2$D or 1α-OHD. Although some patients may experience an initial mild increase in serum alkaline phosphatase, levels of serum alkaline phosphatase progressively decrease with treatment, approaching normal after 6–12 months[170, 172, 173, 178]. The decrease in PTH levels with therapy often corresponds to an increase in serum calcium levels[170, 173]. However, a direct inhibitory role of 1,25$(OH)_2$D on PTH secretion has been shown[15–17, 45, 46]. Whether the levels of 1,25$(OH)_2$D achieved with oral therapy are sufficient to suppress a hyperplastic parathyroid gland remains to be evaluated. However, intravenous 1,25$(OH)_2$D may achieve suppression of PTH independent of the increase in serum calcium[40]. Although the PTH level decreases during most therapeutic trials with 1,25$(OH)_2$D, it rarely becomes normal. This may be secondary both to the fact that metabolites of PTH accumulate in renal failure[63, 179, 180] and, more importantly, involution of hyperplastic parathyroid glands is incomplete[132, 136].

Both radiographical and histological criteria of osteitis fibrosa improve after treatment with 1,25$(OH)_2$D or 1α-OHD. Radiographically, changes of subperiosteal resorption usually improve after 3–12 months of treatment[173, 181–183]. Treatment with 1,25$(OH)_2$D or 1α-OHD is effective therapy for osteitis fibrosa and mixed osteitis fibrosa–osteomalacia. In general, histological improvement includes a decrease in osteoid area, osteoblastic osteoid, osteoclastic resorption, and endosteal fibrosis[170, 172, 174, 183–185]. However, despite treatment the histological abnormalities rarely become normal. In addition, aggressive treatment of patients with severe osteitis fibrosa is often precluded by the development of hypercalcaemia[172, 186]. These patients often require parathyroidectomy.

The vitamin D metabolite, 24,25$(OH)_2$D, has also been used in the treatment of renal osteodystrophy. In the few studies which have evaluated $24,25(OH)_2D$ for the treatment of osteitis fibrosa, no significant effect on serum biochemistry or bone histology was observed[68,187]. Several years ago interest was generated concerning the beneficial effect of $24,25(OH)_2D$ in the treatment of LTOM. After an initial encouraging report[188], subsequent studies have been unable to find a beneficial effect for $24,25(OH)_2D$[65,68].

Treatment of LTOM with vitamin D metabolites has proved, for the most part, to be unrewarding. In one study, LTOM did not improve with 25OHD[169], and, although there have been some reports of clinical improvement with $1,25(OH)_2D$[67,189], for the most part, patients have failed to respond[67,189]. Furthermore, hypercalcaemia has been a major problem during therapy with $1,25(OH)_2D$[67]. The histological findings in LTOM have not changed despite treatment with $1,25(OH)_2D$[65,67]. At the present time, there is no indication to use $1,25(OH)_2D$, or other vitamin D metabolites or analogues, as primary agents in the treatment of LTOM.

The indications for parathyroidectomy must be carefully considered. The operation of choice is either a subtotal parathyroidectomy[190,191] or a total parathyroidectomy with reimplantation of parathyroid tissue in the forearm[192,193]. The decision to perform a parathyroidectomy should be based on histological, radiographical and biochemical confirmation of severe secondary hyperparathyroidism. Findings such as musculoskeletal pain and hypercalcaemia, traditionally ascribed to secondary hyperparathyroidism, are more commonly observed in LTOM[65,67]. In addition, as previously discussed, radiographs may also be misleading[105]. A properly processed bone biopsy is essential to establish the diagnosis securely as well as to provide an index of severity. The PTH level may also be helpful, provided there is a familiarity with usual values in renal failure and proven cases of severe secondary hyperparathyroidism.

In Table 4.3, indications for parathyroidectomy are listed. In all cases, a proven diagnosis, preferably histological, of osteitis fibrosa is essential. In some instances, a trial of $1,25(OH)_2D$ may be warranted. However, in other situations such as the sudden onset of calciphylaxis, parathyroidectomy should be performed promptly[109]. The decision to perform a parathyroidectomy should be made with care, since, in addition to the operative complications, long-term complications have

TABLE 4.3 Indications for parathyroidectomy in patients with renal disease

(1) Patients with renal failure (dialysis dependent) with either an established histological diagnosis of osteitis fibrosa, or a radiographic diagnosis of osteitis fibrosa and biochemical confirmation such as marked elevation of iPTH or serum alkaline phosphatase, who also have at least one of the following problems:

- (a) Persistent hypercalcaemia,
- (b) Progressive or advanced periarticular calcifications,
- (c) Calciphylaxis (ischaemic ulcers or necrosis),
- (d) Progressive or advanced small vessel calcifications,
- (e) Unresponsive pruritus,
- (f) Persistent elevations of serum calcium x phosphorus product (>70 mg/dl), which is resistant to medical management,
- (g) Histological or radiographical affirmation of progressive osteitis fibrosa,
- (h) Rupture of muscle tendonous insertions with little or no trauma.

(2) Renal allograft recipient

- (a) Hypercalcaemia >3.25 mmol/l (13 mg/dl),
- (b) Persistent hypercalcaemia and either:
  - (i) greater than 1 year duration (?)
  - (ii) evidence of deteriorating graft function
  - (iii) renal calculi,
- (c) Suspected primary hyperparathyroidism.

From Felsenfeld and Gutman (1988). 'Parathyroidectomy'. In *Renal Osteodystrophy* (Martinus Nijhoff) In Press

been reported. The possibility has been raised that inadequate parathyroid function may contribute to the development of LTOM. LTOM has been reported in five dialysis patients more than 1 year after parathyroidectomy[194]. In three prospective studies, a bone biopsy was obtained before and 1–3 years after parathyroidectomy[195–197]. Parathyroidectomy resulted in: (1) a decrease in cellular activity, bone resorption and endosteal fibrosis; (2) no increase in osteoid seam width; and (3) a marked decrease in bone formation. Stainable bone aluminium increased significantly after parathyroidectomy in two of the studies[195,197]. Thus, a majority of dialysis patients with osteitis fibrosa developed a state of low bone turnover post-parathyroidectomy. In actuality, this state is not osteomalacia because of the lack of osteoid accumulation. However, it is compatible with the diagnosis of aplastic bone disease. Thus, in summary, although certain definite indications for parathyroidectomy do exist, the decision to perform a parathyroidectomy must be carefully analysed because the reduction of parathyroid hormone by parathyroidectomy may have a harmful effect on bone, especially in the presence of excess aluminium.

The chelating agent, desferrioxamine, has been used for the treatment of LTOM, as well as a test for the diagnosis of LTOM. Desferrioxamine increases aluminium removal via dialysis and thus reduces the burden of aluminium in the body[198,199]. In addition, a recent study has shown that the intraperitoneal administration of desferrioxamine is also an effective means of removing aluminium[200]. Histological studies have shown that desferrioxamine is an effective treatment for aluminium-associated bone disease, both in mixed osteitis fibrosa–osteomalacia[201] and LTOM[202,203]. A more recent study has indicated that desferrioxamine may be effective in LTOM only when PTH increases during treatment[204]. Favourable histological responses were observed in the vast majority of patients with LTOM. The only exceptions were in five patients with a previous parathyroidectomy and one other patient[204]. Consequently, desferrioxamine appears to be an effective treatment for aluminium-associated bone disease, especially in patients with intact parathyroid glands.

The desferrioxamine infusion test has been advocated as a method to diagnose aluminium-associated bone disease. In the test, 40 mg/kg of desferrioxamine is given after haemodialysis and the increment of serum aluminium measured at approximately 40 hours, essentially prior to the next haemodialysis[205–207]. Shorter time intervals have not proved discriminatory[202]. Two studies have found a correlation between the increment in serum aluminium and either stainable bone aluminium[205] or total trabecular bone aluminium[206]. However, others have not found the test to be of diagnostic value[207]. In general, it appears that the bone biopsy remains the only unequivocal method for the diagnosis of aluminium-associated bone disease.

Two other factors which must be considered are oral phosphate binders and the calcium content of the dialysate. In dialysis patients, phosphate retention contributes to the maintenance of secondary hyperparathyroidism and to the deposition of extraosseous calcium deposition. Thus, control of phosphate is important. Conversely, the principal oral phosphate binder, aluminium hydroxide, probably contributes to the development of aluminium-associated bone disease[65,208–210]. At present, there is not an adequate substitute for aluminium hydroxide, but the use of oral calcium carbonate may reduce the amount of aluminium hydroxide necessary to control serum phosphate levels[211–213].

Studies from the early 1970s demonstrated that the calcium content of the dialysate must be greater than 1.5 mmol/l (6 mg/dl) to prevent increases in serum PTH levels[26,214]. At the present time, most haemodialysis units use a dialysate calcium content of 1.5–1.75 mmol/l (6–7 mg/dl). Similarly, calcium losses may be a problem in CAPD, and oral calcium supplementation may be necessary in this population[121–126].

ACKNOWLEDGEMENTS

The authors wish to thank Mrs Charlotte Morris and Mrs Carolyn Clay for secretarial assistance in the preparation of this manuscript.

References

1. Fletcher, H. M. (1911). Case of infantilism with polyuria and chronic renal disease. *Proc. R. Soc. Med.*, **4**, 95–8
2. Parsons, L. J. (1927). The bone changes occurring in renal and coeliac infantilism and the relation to rickets. I. Renal rickets. *Arch. Dis. Child.*, **2**, 1–5
3. Follis, R. H. and Jackson, D. A. (1943). Renal osteomalacia and osteitis fibrosa in adults. *Bull. Johns Hopkins Hosp.*, **72**, 232–6
4. Pappenheimer, A. M. and Wilens, S. L. (1935). Enlargement of the parathyroid glands in renal disease. *Am. J. Pathol.*, **11**, 73–91
5. Pollack, H. and Siegal, S. (1936). Parathyroid hyperplasia and calcinosis associated with renal disease. *J. Mount Sinai Hosp.*, New York, **2**, 270–9
6. Castleman, B. and Mallory, T. B. (1937). Parathyroid hyperplasia in chronic renal insufficiency. *Am. J. Pathol.*, **13**, 553–74

7. Berson, S.A. and Yalow, R.S. (1966). Parathyroid hormone in plasma in adenomatous hyperparathyroidism, uremia, and bronchogenic carcinoma. *Science,* **154,** 907–9
8. Reiss, E., Canterbury, J.M. and Kanter, A. (1969). Circulating parathyroid hormone concentration in chronic renal insufficiency. *Arch. Intern. Med.,* **124,** 417–22
9. Slatopolsky, E., Caglar, S., Pennel, J.P., Taggart, D.D., Canterbury, J.M., Reiss, E. and Bricker, N. (1971). On the pathogenesis of hyperparathyroidism in chronic experimental renal insufficiency in the dog. *J. Clin. Invest.,* **50,** 492–9
10. Slatopolsky, E., Caglar, S., Gradowska, L. *et al.* (1972). On the prevention of secondary hyperparathyroidism in experimental chronic renal disease using 'proportional reduction' of dietary phosphorus intake. *Kidney Int.,* **2,** 147–51
11. Reiss, E., Canterbury, J.M., Bercovitz, M.A. *et al.* (1970). The role of phosphate in the secretion of parathyroid hormone in man. *J. Clin. Invest.,* **49,** 2146–9
12. Goldman, R. and Bassett, S.H. (1954). Phosphorus excretion in renal failure. *J. Clin. Invest.,* **33,** 1623–9
13. Portale, A.A., Booth, B.E., Halloran, B.P. *et al.* (1984). Effect of dietary phosphorus on circulating concentrations of 1,25-dihydroxyvitamin D and immunoreactive parathyroid hormone in children with moderate renal insufficiency. *J. Clin. Invest.,* **73,** 1580–9
14. Llach, F. and Massry, S.G. (1985). On the mechanism of secondary hyperparathyroidism in moderate renal insufficiency. *J. Clin. Endocrinol. Metab.,* **61,** 601–6
15. Cantley, L.K., Russell, J., Lettieri, D. *et al.* (1985). 1,25-dihydroxyvitamin D_3 suppresses parathyroid hormone secretion from bovine parathyroid cells in tissue culture. *Endocrinology,* **117,** 2114–19
16. Silver, J., Naveh-Many, T., Mayer, H. *et al.* (1986). Regulation by vitamin D metabolites of parathyroid hormone gene transcription *in vivo* in the rat. *J. Clin. Invest.,* **78,** 1296–301
17. Lopez-Hilker, S., Galceran, T., Chan, Y.L. *et al.* (1986). Hypocalcemia may not be essential for the development of secondary hyperparathyroidism in chronic renal failure. *J. Clin. Invest.,* **78,** 1097–102
18. Brickman, A.S., Coburn, J.W., Massry, S.G. *et al.* (1974). 1,25-dihydroxyvitamin D_3 in normal man and patients with renal failure. *Ann. Intern. Med.* **80,** 161-8
19. Henderson, R.G., Russell, R.G.G., Ledingham, J.G.G. *et al.* (1974). Effects of 1,25-dihydroxycholecalciferol on calcium absorption, muscle weakness, and bone disease in chronic renal failure. *Lancet,* **1,** 379-84
20. Coburn, J.W., Koppel, M.H., Brickman, A.S. *et al.* (1973). Study of intestinal absorption of calcium in patients with renal failure. *Kidney Int.,* **3,** 264–72
21. Llach, F., Massry, S.G., Singer, F.R. *et al.* (1975). Skeletal resistance of endogeneous parathyroid hormone in patients with early renal failure: a possible cause for secondary hyperparathyroidism. *J. Clin. Endocrinol. Metab.,* **41,** 339–45
22. Wilson, L., Felsenfeld, A., Drezner, M.K. *et al.* (1985). Altered divalent ion metabolism in early renal failure: role of $1,25(OH)_2D$. *Kidney Int.,* **27,** 565–73
23. Portale, A.A., Booth, E.B., Tsai, H.C. *et al.* (1982). Reduced plasma concentration of 1,25-dihydroxyvitamin D in children with moderate renal insufficiency. *Kidney Int.,* **21,** 627–32

24. Adler, A. J., Ferran, N. and Berlyne, G. (1985). Effect of inorganic phospate on serum ionized calcium concentration *in vitro:* a reassessment of the 'trade-off hypothesis'. *Kidney Int.,* **28,** 932–5
25. Fotino, S. (1978). Phosphate excretion in chronic renal failure: evidence for a mechanism other than circulating parathyroid hormone. *Clin. Nephrol.,* **8,** 499–503
26. Fornier, A. E., Arnaud, C. D., Johnson, W. J. *et al.* (1971). Etiology of hyperparathyroidism and bone disease during chronic hemodialysis. II. Factors affecting serum immunoreactive parathyroid hormone. *J. Clin. Invest.,* **50,** 599–616
27. Somerville, P. J. and Kaye, M. (1982). Action of phosphorus on calcium release in isolated perfused rat tails. *Kidney Int.,* **22,** 348–54
28. Kumar, R. (1986). The metabolism and mechanism of action of 1,25-dihydroxyvitamin D_3. *Kidney Int.,* **30,** 793–803
29. Brunette, M. G., Chan, M., Ferriere, C. *et al.* (1978). Site of $1,25(OH)_2$ vitamin D_3 synthesis in the kidney. *Nature (London),* **276,** 287–9
30. Garabedian, N., Holick, M. F., DeLuca, H. F. *et al.* (1972). Control of hydroxycholecalciferol by kidney tissue *in vitro* by calcium. *Nature (London) N. Biol.,* **237,** 63–4
31. Fraser, D. R. and Kodicek, E. (1973). Regulation of 25-hydroxycholecalciferol-1-α hydroxylase activity in kidney by parathyroid hormone. *Nature (London) N. Biol.,* **241,** 163–6
32. Tanaka, Y. and DeLuca, H. F. (1973). The control of 25 hydroxyvitamin D metabolism by inorganic phosphorus. *Arch. Biochem. Biophys.,* **154,** 566–74
33. Gray, R. W., Wilz, D. R., Caldes, A. E. *et al.* (1977). The importance of phosphate in regulating plasma $1,25(OH)_2$-vitamin D levels in humans: studies in healthy subjects, in calcium-stone formers and in patients with primary hyperparathyroidism. *J. Clin. Endocrinol. Metab.,* **45,** 299–306
34. Lund, B. J., Sorenson, O. H., Lund, B. I. *et al.* (1980). Stimulation of 1,25-dihydroxyvitamin D production by parathyroid hormone and hypocalcemia in man. *J. Clin. Endocrinol. Metab.,* **50,** 480–4
35. Trechsel, U., Eisman, J. A., Fischer, J. A. *et al.* (1980). Calcium dependent, parathyroid hormone independent regulation of 1,25 dihydroxyvitamin D. *Am. J. Physiol.,* **239,** E119–24
36. Mason, R. S., Lissner, D., Wilkinson, M. *et al.* (1980). Vitamin D metabolites and their relationship to azotemic osteodystrophy. *Clin. Endocrinol.,* **13,** 375–85
37. Juttman, J. R., Baurman, C. J., De Kam, E. *et al.* (1981). Serum concentrations of metabolites of vitamin D in patients with chronic renal failure. Consequences for the treatment with 1-alpha hydroxy-derivatives. *Clin. Endocrinol.,* **14,** 225–36
38. Slatopolsky, E., Gray, R., Adams, N. D. *et al.* (1978). Low serum levels of $1,25(OH)_2D$ are not responsible for the development of secondary hyperparathyroidism. *Kidney Int.,* **14,** 733 (Abstract)
39. Massry, S. G., Stein, R., Garty, J. *et al.* (1976). Skeletal resistance to the calcemic action of parathyroid hormone in uremia. Role of $1,25(OH)_2D$. *Kidney Int.,* **9,** 467–74
40. Slatopolsky, E., Weerts, C., Thielan, J. *et al.* (1984). Marked suppression of secondary hyperparathyroidism by intravenous administration of 1,25-dihydroxycholecalciferol in uremic patients. *J. Clin. Invest.,* **74,** 2136–43

41. Stanbury, S. W. and Lumb, G. A. (1966). Parathyroid function in chronic renal failure. *Q. J. Med.*, **35**, 1–23
42. Massry, S. G., Coburn, J. W., Lee, D. B. N. *et al.* (1973). Skeletal resistance to parathyroid hormone in renal failure studies in 105 human subjects. *Ann. Intern. Med.*, **78**, 357–64
43. Brown, E. M., Wilkson, R. E., Eastman, R. C. *et al.* (1982). Abnormal regulation of parathyroid hormone release by calcium in secondary hyperparathyroidism due to chronic renal failure. *J. Clin. Endocrinol. Metab.*, **54**, 172–9
44. Bellorin-Font, E., Martin, K., Freitag, J. J. *et al.* (1981). Altered adenylate cyclase kinetics in hyperfunctioning human parathyroid glands. *J. Clin. Endocrinol. Metab.*, **52**, 499–509
45. Chertow, B. S., Baylink, D. J., Wergedal, J. E. *et al.* (1975). Decrease in serum immunoreactive parathyroid hormone in rats and in parathyroid hormone secretion *in vivo* by 1,25 dihydroxycholecalciferol. *J. Clin. Invest.*, **56**, 668–78
46. Chan, Y. L., McKay, C., Dye, E. *et al.* (1986). The effect of 1,25 dihydroxycholecalciferol on parathyroid hormone secretion by monolayer cultures of bovine parathyroid cells. *Calcif. Tissue Int.*, **38**, 27–32
47. Hughes, M. R. and Haussler, M. R. (1978). 1,25 dihydroxycholecalciferol receptors in parathyroid glands. *J. Biol. Chem.*, **253**, 1065–69
48. Wecksler, W. R., Ross, F. P., Mason, R. S. *et al.* (1980). Biochemical properties of the 1,25 dihydroxyvitamin D cytoplasmic receptors from human and chick parathyroid glands. *Arch. Biochem. Biophys.*, **201**, 95–102
49. Silver, J., Russel, J., Lettieri, D. *et al.* (1985). Regulation by vitamin D metabolites of messenger ribonucleic acid for preproparathyroid hormone in isolated bovine parathyroid cells. *Proc. Natl. Acad. Sci. USA.*, **82**, 4270–3
50. Russell, J. E. and Avioli, L. V. (1975). Effect of progressive end-stage renal insufficiency on bone mineral-collagen maturation. *Kidney Int.*, **7**, Suppl. 2, S97–101
51. Alfrey, A. C. and Solomons, C. C. (1976). Bone pyrophosphate in uremia and its association with extraosseous calcification. *J. Clin. Invest.*, **57**, 700–5
52. Burnell, J. M., Teubner, E., Wergedal, J. E. *et al.* (1974). Bone crystal maturation in renal osteodystrophy in humans. *J. Clin. Invest.*, **53**, 52–8
53. Jilka, R. L. (1986). Are osteoblastic cells required for the control of osteoclast activity by parathyroid hormone? *Bone and Mineral,* 1, 261–6
54. Chambers, T. J. (1980). The cellular basis of bone resorption. *Clin. Orthop. Rel. Res.*, **151**, 283–93
55. Parfitt, A. M. and Kleerekoper, M. (1980). The divalent ion homeostatic system: physiology and metabolism of calcium, phosphorus, magnesium, and bone. In Maxwell, M. H. and Kleeman, C. R. (eds.) *Clinical Disorders of Fluid and Electrolyte Metabolism*. pp. 269–398. (McGraw-Hill)
56. Bronner, F. (1982). Calcium homeostasis. In Bronner, F. and Coburn, J. W. (eds.) *Disorders of Mineral Metabolism*. Vol. II, pp. 43–101. (New York: Academic Press)
57. Fallon, M. D. and Teitelbaum, S. L. (1982). The interpretation of fluorescent tetracycline markers in the diagnosis of metabolic bone disease. *Hum. Pathol.*, **13**, 416–17
58. Bordier, P., Marie, P. and Arnaud, C. D. (1975). Evolution of renal osteodystrophy: correlation of bone histomorphometry and serum mineral and immunoreactive parathyroid hormone values before and after treatment with calcium carbonate or 25-hydroxycholecalciferol. *Kidney Int.*, **7**, S102–12

59. Hruska, K. A., Teitelbaum, S. L., Kopelman, R. *et al.* (1978). The predictability of the histologic features of uremic bone disease by non-invasive techniques. *Metab. Bone Rel. Res.*, **1**, 39–44
60. Felsenfeld, A. J., Harrelson, J. M. and Gutman, R. A. (1982). A quantitative histomorphometric comparison of 40 micron thick paragon sections with 5 micron thick Goldner sections in the study of undecalcified bone. *Calif. Tissue Int.*, **34**, 232–8
61. Voigts, A., Felsenfeld, A. J., Andress, D. *et al.* (1984). Parathyroid hormone and bone histology: response to hypocalcemia in osteitis fibrosa. *Kidney Int.*, **25**, 445–52
62. Andress, D. L., Endress, D. B., Maloney, N. A. *et al.* (1986). Comparison of parathyroid hormone assays with bone histomorphometry in renal osteodystrophy. *J. Clin. Endocrinol. Metab.*, **63**, 1163–9
63. Freitag, J., Martin, K. J., Hruska, K. A. *et al.* (1978). Impaired parathyroid hormone metabolism in chronic renal failure. *N. Engl. J. Med.*, **298**, 29–32
64. Malluche, H. H., Ritz, E., Lange, H. P. *et al.* (1976). Bone histology in incipient and advanced renal failure. *Kidney Int.*, **9**, 355–62
65. Llach, F., Felsenfeld, A. J., Coleman, M. D. *et al.* (1986). The natural course of dialysis osteomalacia. *Kidney Int.*, **Suppl. 18**, S74–9
66. Bordier, P. J., Tun-Chot, S., Eastwood, J. B. *et al.* (1973). Lack of histological evidence of vitamin D abnormality in the bones of anephric patients. *Clin. Sci.*, **44**, 33–41
67. Hodsman, A. B., Sherrard, D. J., Wong, E. G. C. *et al.* (1981). Vitamin D resistant osteomalacia on hemodialysis patients lacking secondary hyperparathyroidism: description of the syndrome in 19 patients. *Ann. Intern. Med.* **94**, 629–37
68. Dunstan, C. R., Hills, E., Norman, A. A. *et al.* (1985). Treatment of hemodialysis bone disease with $24,25\text{-}(OH)_2D_3$ and $1,25\text{-}(OH)_2D_3$ alone or in combination. *Mineral Electrolyte Metab.*, **11**, 358–68
69. Massry, S. G., Goldstein, D. A. and Malluche, H. H. (1980). Current status of the use of $1,25(OH)_2D_3$ in the management of renal osteodystrophy. *Kidney Int.*, **18**, 409–18
70. Johnson, W. J. (1986). Use of vitamin D analogs in renal osteodystrophy. *Sem. Nephrol.*, **6**, 31–41
71. Platts, M. M., Goode, G. C. and Hislop, J. S. (1977). Composition of water supply and the incidence of fractures and encephalopathy in patients on home dialysis. *Br. Med. J.*, **2**, 657–60
72. Ward, M. K., Feest, T. G., Ellis, H. A. *et al.* (1978). Osteomalacic dialysis: evidence for a water-borne aetiological agent, probably aluminium. *Lancet*, **1**, 841–5
73. Parkinson, I. S., Feest, T. G., Ward, M. K. *et al.* (1979). Fracturing dialysis osteodystrophy and dialysis encephalopathy: an epidemiological survey. *Lancet*, **1**, 406–9
74. Parkinson, I. S., Ward, M. K. and Kerr, D. N. S. (1981). Dialysis encephalopathy, bone disease and anaemia: The aluminium intoxication syndrome during regular haemodialysis. *J. Clin. Pathol.*, **34**, 1285–94
75. Ellis, H. A., McCarthy, J. H. and Herrington, J. (1979). Bone aluminium in hemodialysed patients and in rats injected with aluminium chloride: relationship to impaired bone mineralization. *J. Clin. Pathol.*, **32**, 832–44
76. Robertson, J. A., Felsenfeld, A. J., Haygood, C. G. *et al.* (1983). An animal

model of aluminium-induced osteomalacia: role of chronic renal failure. *Kidney Int.*, **23**, 327–35
77. Maloney, N. A., Ott, S., Alfrey, A. C. *et al.* (1982). Histologic quantitation of aluminium in iliac bone from patients with renal failure. *J. Lab. Clin. Med.*, **99**, 206–16
78. Malluche, H. H., Smith, A. J., Abreo, K. *et al.* (1984). The use of desferrioxamine in the management of bone aluminium accumulation in patients with renal failure. *N. Engl. J. Med.*, **311**, 140–4
79. Ott, S. M., Andress, D. L., Nebeker, H. G. *et al.* (1986). Changes in bone histology after treatment with desferrioxamine. *Kidney Int.*, **29**, (Suppl 18), S108–13
80. Ihle, B. U., Cochran, M., Becker, G. *et al.* (1984). Bone 'buffering' capacity in aluminium associated bone disease. *Kidney Int.*, **26**, 234 (Abstract)
81. Rodriguez, M., Felsenfeld, A. and Llach, F. (1987). The role of aluminium in the development of hypercalcemia in the rat. *Kidney Int.*, **31**, 766–71
82. Lorenzo, V., Rodriguez, M., Felsenfeld, A. *et al.* (1986). Aluminium toxicity in parathyroidectomized rats resembles aplastic bone disease. *Kidney Int.*, **29**, 164 (Abstract)
83. Rodriguez, M., Felsenfeld, A. and Llach, F. (1986). Transplanted parathyroid glands function despite aluminium exposure. *Kidney Int.*, **29**, 170 (Abstract)
84. Henry, D. A., Goodman, W. G., Nudelman, R. K. *et al.* (1984). Parenteral aluminium administration in the dog. I. Plasma kinetics, tissue levels, calcium metabolism and parathyroid hormone. *Kidney Int.*, **25**, 362–9
85. Andress, D., Felsenfeld, A. J., Voigts, A. *et al.* (1983). Parathyroid hormone response to hypocalcemia in hemodialysis patients with osteomalacia. *Kidney Int.*, **24**, 364–70
86. Kraut, J. A., Shinaberger, J. H., Singer, F. R. *et al.* (1983). Parathyroid gland responsiveness to acute hypocalcemia in hemodialysis patients with osteomalacia. *Kidney Int.*, **23**, 725–30
87. Morrisey, J. and Slatopolsky, E. (1986). Effect of aluminium on parathyroid hormone secretion. *Kidney Int.*, **29**, (Suppl 18), S41–4
88. Bourdeau, A. M., Plachot, J. J., Cournot-Witmer, G. *et al.* (1987). Parathyroid response to aluminium *in vitro:* ultrastructural changes and PTH release. *Kidney Int.*, **31**, 15–24
89. Cournot-Witmer, G., Zingraff, J., Plachot, J. J. *et al.* (1981). Aluminium localization in bone from hemodialyzed patients: relationship to matrix mineralization. *Kidney Int.*, **20**, 375–81
90. Plachot, J. J., Cournot-Witmer, G., Halpern, S. *et al.* (1984). Bone ultrastructure and X-ray microanalysis of aluminium-intoxicated hemodialyzed patients. *Kidney Int.*, **25**, 796–803
91. Charhon, S. A., Chavassieux, P. M., Chapuy, M. C. *et al.* (1985). Low rate of bone formation with or without histologic appearance of osteomalacia in patients with aluminium intoxication. *J. Lab. Clin. Med.*, **106**, 123–31
92. Alvarez-Ude, F., Feest, T. G., Ward, M. K. *et al.* (1978). Hemodialysis bone disease: correlation between clinical, histologic, and other findings. *Kidney Int.*, **14**, 68–73
93. Chan, Y. L., Furlong, T. J., Cornish, C. J. *et al.* (1985). Dialysis osteodystrophy: a study involving 94 patients. *Medicine*, **64**, 296–309
94. Evans, R. A., Flynn, J., Dunstan, C. R. *et al.* (1982). Bone metabolism in chronic renal failure. *Mineral Electrolyte Metab.*, **7**, 207–18

95. Ritz, E., Malluche, H. H., Bonner, J. *et al.* (1974). Metabolic bone disease in patients on maintenance hemodialysis. *Nephron.*, **12,** 393–404
96. Pierides, A. M., Skillen, A. W. and Ellis, H. A. (1979). Serum alkaline phosphatase in azotemic and hemodialysis osteodystrophy: a study of isoenzyme patterns, their correlation with bone histology, and their changes in response to treatment with $1\alpha(OH)D_3$ and $1,25(OH)_2D_3$. *J. Lab. Clin. Med.*, **93,** 899–909
97. Hodsman, A. B., Sherrard, D. J., Alfrey, A. *et al.* (1982). Bone aluminium and histomorphometric features of renal osteodystrophy. *J. Clin. Endocrinol. Metab.*, **54,** 539–46
98. Malluche, H. H., Faugere, M. C., Fanti, P. *et al.* (1984). Plasma levels of bone Gla-protein reflect bone formation in patients on chronic maintenance dialysis. *Kidney Int.*, **26,** 869–74
99. Gundberg, C. M. and Weinstein, R. S. (1986). Multiple immunoreactive forms of osteocalcin in serum. *J. Clin. Invest.*, **77,** 1762–7
100. Dent, C. E. and Hodson, C. J. (1954). Radiological changes associated with certain metabolic bone diseases. *Br. J. Radiol.*, **27,** 605–22
101. Meema, H. E., Rabinovich, S., Meema, S. *et al.* (1972). Improved radiological diagnosis of azotemic osteodystrophy. *Radiology,* **102,** 1–10
102. Meema, H. E., Merndok, H. and Oreopoulos, D. G. (1983). Radiology of renal osteodystrophy. In Brenner, B. M. and Stein, J. H. (eds.) *Divalent Ion Homeostasis, Contemporary Issues in Nephrology.* Vol. II, pp. 261–89. (Edinburgh: Churchill Livingstone)
103. Ritz, E., Prager, P., Krempien, B. *et al.* (1978). Skeletal X-ray findings and bone histology in patients on hemodialysis. *Kidney Int.*, **13,** 316–23
104. Debnern, J. W., Bates, M. L., Kopelman, R. C. *et al.* (1977). Radiological, pathological correlations in uremic bone disease. *Radiology,* **125,** 653–8
105. Sherrard, D. J., Ott, S. M. and Andress, D. L. (1985). Pseudohyperparathyroidism syndrome associated with aluminium intoxication in patients with renal failure. *Am. J. Med.*, **79,** 127–30
106. Coburn, J. W. and Slatopolsky, E. (1986). Vitamin D, parathyroid hormone, and renal osteodystrophy. In Brenner, B. M. and Rector Jr, F. C. (eds.). *The Kidney.* 3rd edn., pp. 1657–729. (W. B. Saunders)
107. Karsenty, G., Vigneron, N., Jorgetti, V. *et al.* (1986). Value of the ^{99m}Tc-methylene diphosphonate bone scan in renal osteodystrophy. *Kidney Int.*, **29,** 1058–65
108. Hodson, E. M., Howman-Giles, R. B., Evans, R. A. *et al.* (1981). The diagnosis of renal osteodystrophy: a comparison of Technetium-99m-pyrophosphate bone scintigraphy with other techniques. *Clin. Nephrol.*, **16,** 24–8
109. Gipstein, R. M., Coburn, J. W., Adams, D. A. *et al.* (1976). A syndrome of tissue necrosis and vascular calcification in 11 patients with chronic renal failure. *Arch. Intern. Med.*, **136,** 1273–80
110. Anderson, H. C. (1983). Calcific diseases. *Arch. Pathol. Lab. Med.*, **107,** 341–8
111. Contiguglia, S., Alfrey, A. C., Miller, N. L. *et al.* (1973). Nature of soft tissue calcification in uremia. *Kidney Int.*, **4,** 229–35
112. LeGeros, R. Z., Contiguglia, S. R. and Alfrey, A. C. (1973). Pathological calcifications associated with uremia: two types of calcium phosphate deposits. *Calc. Tiss. Res.*, **13,** 173–85
113. Ibels, L. S., Alfrey, A. C., Huffer, W. E., *et al.* (1979). Arterial calcification and pathology in uremic patients undergoing dialysis. *Am. J. Med.*, **66,** 790–6

114. Jacobs, L. J., Manten, H., Myerburg, R. J., *et al.* (1979). Pseudohypertension due to diffuse vascular calcification in chronic renal failure. *Ann. Intern. Med.*, **90**, 353–4
115. Conger, J. D., Hammond, W. S., Alfrey, A. C., *et al.* (1975). Pulmonary calcification in chronic dialysis patients: Clinical and pathologic studies. *Ann. Intern. Med.*, 330–6
116. Dreher, W. and Shelp, W. (1975). Atrioventricular block in a long term dialysis patient. Reversal after parathyroidectomy. *J. Am. Med. Assoc.*, **234**, 954–5
117. Parfitt, A. M. (1969). Soft tissue calcification in uremia. *Arch. Intern. Med.*, **124**, 544–56
118. Massry, S. G., Popovtzer, M. M., Coburn, J. W., *et al.* (1968). Intractable pruritus as a manifestation of 2° hyperparathyroidism in uremia. Disappearance of itching following subtotal parathyroidectomy. *N. Engl. J. Med.*, **279**, 697–700
119. Kraikitpanitch, S., Lindeman, R. D., Yunice, A., *et al.* (1978). Effect of azotemia on the myocardial accumulation of calcium. *Mineral Electrolyte Metab.*, **1**, 12–20
120. Ejerblad, S., Eriksson, I. and Johansson, H. (1979). An experimental study with special reference to the effect of parathyroidectomy. *Scand. J. Urol. Nephrol.*, **13**, 161–9
121. Gokal, R., Ramos, J. M., Ellis, H. A. *et al.* (1983). Histological renal osteodystrophy, and 25 hydroxycholecalciferol and aluminium levels in patients on continuous ambulatory peritoneal dialysis. *Kidney Int.*, **23**, 15–21
122. Digenis, C., Khanna, R., Pierratos, A. *et al.* (1983). Renal osteodystrophy in patients maintained on CAPD for more than three years., *Peritoneal Dial. Bull.*, **3**, 81–6
123. Zucchelli, P., Catizone, L., Casanova, S. *et al.* (1984). Renal osteodystrophy in CAPD patients. *Mineral Electrolyte Metab.*, **10**, 326–32
124. Delmez, J. A., Fallon, M. D., Bergfeld, M. A. *et al.* (1986). Continuous ambulatory peritoneal dialysis and bone. *Kidney Int.*, **30**, 379–84
125. Tielemans, C., Aubry, C. and Dratwa, M. (1981). The effect of continuous ambulatory peritoneal dialysis (CAPD) on renal osteodystrophy. In Gahl, G. M., Kessel, M. and Nolph, K. D. (eds.) *Proceedings of the 2nd International Symposium of Peritoneal Dialysis.* pp. 455–60. (Berlin: Excerpta Medica)
126. Pederson, J. A., Felsenfeld, A. J., Voigts, A. L. *et al.* (1986). Effects of CAPD on renal osteodystrophy in unmodified patients moving from hemodialysis to CAPD. In *Frontiers in Peritoneal Dialysis.* pp. 471–7. (New York: Field, Rich and Associates, Inc.)
127. Lund, B., Clausen, E., Friedberg, M. *et al.* (1980). Serum 1,25-dihydroxycholecalciferol in anephric, haemodialyzed and kidney-transplanted patients. *Nephron*, **25**, 30–3
128. Garabedian, M., Silve, C., Levy-Bentolila, D. *et al.* (1981). Changes in plasma 1,25 and 24,25-dihydroxyvitamin D after renal transplantation in children. *Kidney Int.*, **20**, 403–10
129. David, D. S., Sakai, S., Brennan, B. L. *et al.* (1973). Hypercalcemia after renal transplantation: long-term follow-up data. *N. Engl. J. Med.*, **289**, 398–401
130. Pletka, P. G., Strom, T. B., Hampers, C. L. *et al.* (1976). Secondary hyperparathyroidism in human kidney transplant recipients. *Nephron*, **17**, 371–81
131. Conceicao, S. C., Wilkinson, R., Feest, T. G. *et al.* (1981). Hypercalcemia following renal transplantation: causes and consequences. *Clin. Nephrol.*, **16**, 235–44

132. McCarron, D. A., Muther, R. S., Lenfesty, B. *et al.* (1982). Parathyroid function in persistent hyperparathyroidism: relationship to gland size. *Kidney Int.*, **22,** 662–70
133. Cundy, T., Kanis, J. A., Heynen, G. *et al.* Calcium metabolism and hyperparathyroidism after renal transplantation. *Q. J. Med.*, **52,** 67–78
134. Rosenbaum, R. W., Hruska, K. A., Korkor, A. *et al.* (1981). Decreased phosphate reabsorption after renal transplantation: evidence for a mechanism independent of calcium and parathyroid hormone. *Kidney Int.*, **19,** 568–78
135. Better, O. S. (1980). Tubular dysfunction following kidney transplantation. *Nephron.*, **25,** 209–13
136. Parfitt, A. M. (1982). Hypercalcemic hyperparathyroidism following renal transplantation: differential diagnosis, management, and implications for cell population control in the parathyroid gland. *Mineral Electrolyte Metab.*, **8,** 92–112
137. Ihle, B. U., Buchanan., M. R. C., Stevens, B. *et al.* (1982). The efficacy of various treatment modalities on aluminium associated bone disease. *Proc. Eur. Dial. Transplant Assoc.*, **19,** 195–201
138. Podenphant, J., Salem, N., Sypitkowski, C. *et al.* (1985). Reversal of aluminium related dialysis osteomalacia after transplantation. *Bone*, **6,** 405 (Abstract)
139. Parfitt, A. M. (1986). Are bone problems of dialysis patients always solved by renal transplantation? *Cases in Metabolic Bone Disease*, **1,** No. 4. (New York: Medical Projects, Inc.)
140. Moorehead, J. F., Wills, M. R., Ahmed, K. Y. *et al.* (1974). Hypophosphatemic osteomalacia after cadaveric renal transplantation. *Lancet*, **1,** 694–7
141. Felsenfeld, A. J., Gutman, R. A., Drezner, M. *et al.* (1986). Hypophosphatemia in long-term renal transplant recipients: effects on bone histology and 1,25-dihydroxycholecalciferol. *Mineral Electrolyte Metab.*, **12,** 333–41
142. Bewick, M., Stewart, P. H., Rudge, C. *et al.* (1976). Avascular necrosis of bone in patients undergoing renal allotransplantation. *Clin. Nephrol.*, **5,** 66–72
143. Hawking, K. M. (1976). Avascular necrosis of bone after renal transplantation. *N. Engl. J. Med.*, **294,** 397
144. Ibel, L. S., Alfrey, A. C., Huffer, W. E. *et al.* (1978). Aseptic necrosis of bone following renal transplantation: experience of 194 transplant recipients and review of the literature. *Medicine*, **57,** 25–45
145. Glimcher, M. G. and Kenzora, J. E. (1979). The biology of osteonecrosis of the human femoral head and its clinical implications. I. Tissue biology. *Clin. Orthop.*, **138,** 284–309
146. Glimcher, M. G. and Kenzora, J. E (1979). The biology of osteonecrosis of the human femoral head and its clinical implications. II. The pathological changes in the femoral head as an organ and in the hip joint. *Clin. Orthop.*, **139,** 283–312
147. Glimcher, M. G. and Kenzora, J. E. (1979). The biology of osteonecrosis of the human femoral head and its clinical implications. III. Discussion of the etiology and genesis of the pathological sequelae: comments on treatment. *Clin. Orthop.*, **140,** 273–312
148. Creuss, R. L. (1986). Osteonecrosis of bone: current concepts as to etiology and pathogenesis. *Clin. Orthop.*, **208,** 30–9
149. Ficat, R. P. (1985). Idiopathic bone necrosis of the femoral head: early diagnosis and treatment. *Bone Joint Surg.* (British), **67,** 3–9
150. Hungerford, D. S. (1981). Pathogenetic considerations in ischemic necrosis of bone. *Can. J. Surg.*, **24,** 583–8

151. Nixon, J. E. (1983). Avascular necrosis of bone: a review. *J. R. Soc. Med.*, **76,** 681–92
152. Frost, H. M. (1964). The etiodynamics of aseptic necrosis of the femoral head. In Proceedings of the *Conference on Aseptic Necrosis of the Femoral Head.* (Reynolds, F. C., Chairman). p. 393. St Louis, Missouri
153. Arlot, M. E., Bonjean, M., Chavassieux, P. *et al.* (1983). Bone histology in adults with aseptic necrosis. *J. Bone Joint Surg.* (*American*), **65A,** 1319–27
154. Pierides, A. M., Simpson, W., Stainsby, D. *et al.* (1975). Avascular necrosis of bone following renal transplantation. *Q. J. Med.*, **44,** 459–80
155. Elmstedt, E. (1981). Skeletal complications in the renal transplant recipient. *Acta Orthop. Scand.*, **52,** (Suppl 190), 7–44
156. Briggs, W. A., Hampers, C. L. O., Merill, J. P. *et al.* (1972). Aseptic necrosis in the femur after renal transplantation. *Ann. Surg.*, **175,** 282–9
157. Potter, D. E., Genant, H. K. and Salvatierra, O. (1978). Avascular necrosis of bone after renal transplantation. *Am. J. Dis. Child.*, **132,** 1125–9
158. Conklin, J. J., Alderson, P. O., Zizic, T. M. *et al.* (1983). Comparison of bone scan and radiograph sensitivity in the detection of steroid-induced ischemic necrosis of bone. *Radiology*, **147,** 221–6
159. Gillespy III, T., Genant, H. K. and Helms, C. A. (1986). Magnetic resonance imaging of osteonecrosis. *Radiol. Clin. N. Am.*, **24,** 193–208
160. Collier, B. D., Carrera, G. F., Johnson, R. P. *et al.* (1985). Detection of femoral head avascular necrosis in adults by SPECT. *J. Nucl. Med.*, **26,** 979–87
161. Stanbury, S. W. and Lumb, G. A. (1962). Metabolic studies of renal osteodystrophy. I. Calcium, phosphorus, and nitrogen metabolism in rickets, osteomalacia, and hyperparathyroidism complicating chronic uremia and in the osteomalacia of the adult Fanconi syndrome. *Medicine*, **41,** 1–30
162. Verbeckmoes, R., Bouillon, R. and Krempien, B. (1973). Osteodystrophy of dialysed patients treated with vitamin D. *Proc. Eur. Dial. Transplant. Assoc.*, **10,** 217–25
163. Voigts, A. L., Felsenfeld, A. J. and Llach, F. (1983). The effect of calciferol and its metabolites on patients with chronic renal failure. I. Calciferol, dihydrotachysterol, and calcifediol. *Arch. Intern. Med.*, **143,** 960–3
164. Liu, S. H. and Chu, H. I. (1943). Studies of calcium and phosphorus metabolism with special reference to pathogenesis and effects of dihydrotachysterol (ATIO) and iron. *Medicine*, **22,** 103–61
165. Kaye, M., Chatterjee, G., Cohen, G. F. *et al.* (1970). Arrest of hyperparathyroid bone disease with dihydrotachysterol in patients undergoing chronic hemodialysis. *Ann. Intern. Med.*, **73,** 225–33
166. Cordy, P. E. and Mills, D. M. (1981). The early detection and treatment of renal osteodystrophy. *Mineral Electrolyte Metab.*, **5,** 311–20
167. Smith, J. E. and Goodman, D. S. (1979). The turnover and transport of vitamin D and of a polar metabolite with the properties of 25-hydroxycholecalciferol in human plasma. *J. Clin. Invest.*, **50,** 2159–65
168. Recker, R., Schoenfeld, P., Letteri, J. *et al.* (1978). The efficacy of calcifediol in renal osteodystrophy. *Arch. Intern. Med.*, **138,** 857–63
169. Frost, H. M., Griffith, D. L., Jee, W. S. S. *et al.* (1981). Histomorphometric changes in trabecular bone of renal failure patients treated with calcifediol. *Metabol. Bone Dis. Rel. Res.*, **2,** 285–95
170. Pierides, A. M., Simpson, W., Ward, M. K. *et al.* (1976). Variable response to

long-term 1α-hydroxycholecalciferol in hemodialysis osteodystrophy. *Lancet*, **1**, 1092–5

171. Madsen, S. and Olgaard, K. (1976). 1α-hydroxycholecalciferol treatment of adults with chronic renal failure. *Acta Med. Scand.*, **200**, 1–5
172. Kanis, J. A., Cundy, T., Earnshaw, M. *et al.* (1979). Treatment of renal bone disease with 1α-hydroxylated derivatives of vitamin D_3. *Q. J. Med.*, **48**, 289–322
173. Goldstein, D. A., Malluche, H. H. and Massry, S. G. (1979). Management of renal osteodystrophy with $1,25(OH)_2D_3$. I. Effects on clinical, radiographic, and biochemical parameters. *Mineral Electrolyte Metab.*, **2**, 35–47
174. Malluche, H. H., Goldstein, D. A. and Massry, S. G. (1979). Management of renal osteodystrophy with $1,25(OH)_2D_3$. II. Effect on histopathology of bone: evidence for healing of osteomalacia. *Mineral Electrolyte Metab.*, **2**, 48–55
175. Winkler, S. N., Brickman, A. S., Wong, E. G. C *et al.* (1979). Hypercalcemia during treatment of uremic patients with $1,25(OH)_2D_3$: analysis of 43 cases. In Norman, A. W., Schaeffer, K. and Herrath, D. U. (eds.) *Vitamin D Basic Research and Its Clinical Application.* pp. 851–2. (Berlin, Walter de Gruyter and Company)
176. Memmos, D. E., Eastwood, J. B., Talner, L. B. *et al.* (1981). Double-blind trial of oral 1,25-dihydroxyvitamin D_3 versus placebo in asymptomatic hyperparathyroidism in patients receiving maintenance hemodialysis. *Br. Med. J.*, **282**, 1919–24
177. Voigts, A. L., Felsenfeld, A. J. and Llach, F. (1983). The effects of calciferol and its metabolites on patients with chronic renal failure. II. Calcitriol, 1α-hydroxyvitamin D_3, and 24,25-dihydroxyvitamin D_3. *Arch. Intern. Med.*, **143**, 1205–11
178. Davie, M. W. J., Chalmers, T. M., Hunter, J. O. *et al.* (1976). Alpha hydroxycholecalciferol in chronic renal failure: studies of the effect of oral doses. *Ann. Intern. Med.*, **84**, 281–5
179. Hruska, K. A., Kopelman, R., Rutherford, R. *et al.* (1975). Metabolism of immunoreactive parathyroid hormone in the dog. The role of the kidney and the effects of chronic renal disease. *J. Clin. Invest.*, **56**, 39–48
180. Martin, K. J., Hruska, K. A., Lewis, J. *et al.* (1977). The renal handling of parathyroid hormone. Role of peritubular uptake and glomerular filtration. *J. Clin. Invest.*, **60**, 808–16
181. Henderson, R. G., Ledingham, J. G. G., Oliver, D. O. *et al.* (1974). Effects of 1,25 dihydroxycholecalciferol on calcium absorption, muscle weakness, and bone disease in chronic renal failure. *Lancet*, **1**, 379–84
182. Chan, J. C. N., Oldham, S. B., Holick, M. F. *et al.* (1975). 1α-hydroxyvitamin D_3 in chronic renal failure. A potent analogue of the kidney hormone 1,25-dihydroxycholecalciferol. *J. Am. Med. Assoc.*, **234**, 47–52
183. Nielsen, H. E., Melsen, F., Christiansen, M. S. *et al.* (1977). 1α-hydroxycholecalciferol treatment of long-term hemodialyzed patients. Effects on mineral metabolism, bone mineral content, and bone morphometry. *Clin. Nephrol.*, **8**, 429–34
184. Ellis, H. A., Pierides, A. M., Feest, T. G. *et al.* (1977). Histopathology of renal osteodystrophy with particular reference to the effects of 1α-hydroxyvitamin D_3 in patients treated by long-term hemodialysis. *Clin. Endocrinol.*, **7** (Suppl), 31–8
185. Valentzas, C., Oreopoulos, D. G., Pierratos, A. *et al.* (1981). Treatment of renal

osteodystrophy with 1,25-dihydroxycholecalciferol. *Can. Med. Assoc. J.*, **124,** 577–83
186. Prior, J. C., Cameron, E. C., Ballon, H. S. *et al.* (1979). Experience with 1,25-dihydroxycholecalciferol therapy in patients undergoing hemodialysis with progressive vitamin D_2-treated osteodystrophy. *Am. J. Med.*, **67,** 583–9
187. Muirhead, N., Catto, G. R. D., Edward, N. *et al.* (1980). Comparison of $1,25(OH)_2D_3$ and $24,25(OH)_2D_3$ in the long-term treatment of renal osteodystrophy. *Proc. Eur. Dial. Transplant Assoc.*, **17,** 543–7
188. Hodsman, A. B., Wong, E. G. C., Sherrard, D. J. *et al.* (1983). Preliminary trials with 24,25 dihydroxyvitamin D_3 in dialysis osteomalacia. *Am. J. Med.*, **74,** 407–14
189. Coburn, J. W., Sherrard, D. J., Brickman, A. S. *et al.* (1980). A skeletal mineralizing defect in dialysis patients: a syndrome resembling osteomalacia but unrelated to vitamin D. *Contrib. Nephrol.*, **18,** 172–83
190. Gordon, H. E., Coburn, J. W. and Passaro, E. (1972). Surgical management of secondary hyperparathyroidism. *Arch. Surg.*, **104,** 520–6
191. Kuhlback, B., Sivula, A., Koch, B. *et al.* (1977). Secondary hyperparathyroidism and parathyroidectomy in terminal chronic renal failure. *Scand. J. Urol. Nephrol.*, **42** (Suppl), 140–3
192. Wells, S. A., Ellis, G. J., Gunnells, J. C. *et al.* (1976). Parathyroid autotransplantation in primary parathyroid hyperplasia. *N. Eng. J. Med.*, **295,** 57–62
193. DuBost, C. L., Drueke, T., Jeaneau, P. L. *et al.* (1980). Hyperparathyroidie secondaire: parathyroidectomie subtotale on totale avec autotransplantation parathyroidienne. *Nouv. Presse Med.*, **9,** 2709–13
194. Felsenfeld, A. J., Harrelson, J. M., Gutman, R. A. *et al.* (1982). Osteomalacia after parathyroidectomy in patients with uremia. *Ann. Intern. Med.*, **96,** 34–9
195. Andress, D. L., Ott, S. M., Malony, N. A. *et al.* (1985). Effect of parathyroidectomy on bone aluminium accumulation in chronic renal failure. *N. Engl. J. Med.*, **312,** 468–73
196. Charhon, S. A., Berland, Y. R., Olmer, M. J. *et al.* (1985). Effects of parathyroidectomy on bone formation and mineralization in hemodialyzed patients. *Kidney Int.*, **27,** 426–35
197. De Vernejoul, M. C., Marchais, S., London, G. *et al.* (1985). Increased bone aluminium deposition after subtotal parathyroidectomy in dialyzed patients. *Kidney Int.*, **27,** 785–91
198. Chang, T. M. S. and Barre, P. (1983). Effect of desferrioxamine on removal of aluminium and iron by coated charcoal haemoperfusion and haemodialysis. *Lancet*,, **2,** 1051–3
199. Stummroll, H. K., Graf, H. and Meisinger, V. (1984). Effect of desferrioxamine on aluminium kinetics during hemodialysis. *Mineral Electrolyte Metab.*, **10,** 263–6
200. Hercz, G., Salusky, I. B., Norris, K. C. *et al.* (1986). Aluminium removal by peritoneal dialysis: intravenous vs intraperitoneal deferoxamine. *Kidney Int.*, **30,** 944–8
201. Malluche, H. H., Smith, A. J., Abreo, K. *et al.* (1984). The use of deferoxamine in the management of aluminium accumulation in bone in patients with renal failure. *N. Engl. J. Med.*, **311,** 140–4

202. Brown, D. J., Dawborn, J. K., Ham. K. N. *et al.* (1982). Treatment of dialysis osteomalacia with desferrioxamine. *Lancet.*, **2,** 343–5
203. Ott, S. M., Andress, D. L., Nebeker, H. G. *et al.* (1986). Changes in bone histology after treatment with desferrioxamine. *Kidney Int.*, **29** Suppl 18, S108–13
204. Andress, D. L., Nebeker, H. G., Ott, S. M. *et al.* (1987). Bone histologic response to long-term deferoxamine and aluminium bone disease. *Kidney Int.*, **31,** 1344–50
205. Milliner, D. S., Nebeker, H. G., Ott, S. M. *et al.* (1984). Use of deferoxamine infusion test in the diagnosis of aluminium-related osteodystrophy. *Ann. Intern. Med.*, **101,** 755–80
206. Berland, Y., Charhon, S. A., Olmer, M. *et al.* (1985). Predictive value of desferrioxamine infusion test for bone aluminium deposits in hemodialyzed patients. *Nephron*, **40,** 433–5
207. Hodsman, A. B., Hood, S. A., Brown, P. *et al.* (1985). Do serum aluminium levels reflect underlying skeletal aluminium accumulation and bone histology before or after chelation by deferoxamine? *J. Lab. Clin. Med.*, **106,** 674–81
208. Felsenfeld, A. J., Gutman, R. A., Llach, F. *et al.* (1982). Osteomalacia in chronic renal failure: a syndrome previously reported only with maintenance dialysis. *Am. J. Nephrol.*, **2,** 147–54
209. Andreoli, S. P., Bergstein, J. M. and Sherrard, D. J. (1984). Aluminium intoxication in nondialyzed azotemic children from aluminium containing phosphate binders. *N. Eng. J. Med.*, **310,** 1079–84
210. Kaye, M. (1983). Oral aluminium toxicity in a non-dialyzed patient with renal failure. *Clin. Nephrol.*, **20,** 208–16
211. Moriniere, P. H., Roussel, A., Tahiri, Y. *et al.* (1982). Substitution of aluminium hydroxide by high doses of calcium carbonate in patients on chronic hemodialysis: disappearance of hyperaluminaemia and equal control of hyperparathyroidism. *Proc. Eur. Dial. Transplant. Assoc.*, **19,** 784–7
212. Slatopolsky, E., Weerts, C., Lopez-Hilker, S.. *et al.* (1986). Calcium carbonate as a phosphate binder in patients with chronic renal failure undergoing dialysis. *N. Engl. J. Med.*, **315,** 157–61
213. Fornier, A., Moriniere, P., Sebert, J. L. *et al.* (1986). Calcium carbonate, an aluminium-free agent for control of hyperphosphatemia, hypocalcemia, and hyperparathyroidism in uremia. *Kidney Int.*, **29** (Suppl 18), S114–19
214. Johnson, W. J., Goldsmith, R. S. and Arnaud, C. D. (1972). Prevention and treatment of progressive secondary hyperparathyroidism in advanced renal failure. *Med. Clin. N. Am.*, **56,** 961–75

INDEX

GPSR Compliance

The European Union's (EU) General Product Safety Regulation (GPSR) is a set of rules that requires consumer products to be safe and our obligations to ensure this.

If you have any concerns about our products, you can contact us on ProductSafety@springernature.com

In case Publisher is established outside the EU, the EU authorized representative is:

Springer Nature Customer Service Center GmbH
Europaplatz 3
69115 Heidelberg, Germany

Batch number: 10761599

Printed by Printforce, the Netherlands